thefacts

Post-traumatic stress

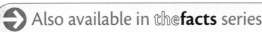# Also available in the**facts** series

ADHD: the**facts**
SECOND EDITION
Selikowitz

Alcoholism: the**facts**
FOURTH EDITION
Manzardo et al.

Asthma: the**facts**
Arshad and Babu

Autism and Asperger Syndrome: the**facts**
Baron-Cohen

Back Pain: the**facts**
Lee

Borderline Personality Disorder: the**facts**
Krawitz and Jackson

Breast Cancer: the**facts**
Saunders

Chronic Fatigue Syndrome: the**facts**
SECOND EDITION
Campling and Sharpe

Chronic Obstructive Pulmonary Disease (COPD):
the**facts**
Currie

Cosmetic Surgery: the**facts**
Waterhouse

Cystic Fibrosis: the**facts**
FOURTH EDITION
Thompson and Harris

Diabetes: the**facts**
Matthews et al.

Down Syndrome: the**facts**
THIRD EDITION
Selikowitz

Eating Disorders: the**facts**
SIXTH EDITION
Abraham

Epilepsy: the**facts**
THIRD EDITION
Appleton and Marson

Epilepsy in Women: the**facts**
Betts and Clarke

Falls: the**facts**
Darowski

Head Injury: the**facts**
Daisley, Tams, and Kischka

Huntington's Disease: the**facts**
SECOND EDITION
Quarrell

Infertility: the**facts**
Davies, Overton, and Webber

Inflammatory Bowel Disease: the**facts**
Langmead and Irving

Insomnia and other Adult Sleep Problems:
the**facts**
Stores

Lung Cancer: the**facts**
THIRD EDITION
Falk and Williams

Lupus: the**facts**
SECOND EDITION
Isenberg and Manzi

Motor Neuron Disease: the**facts**
Talbot and Marsden

Muscular Dystrophy: the**facts**
THIRD EDITION
Emery

Myotonic Dystrophy: the**facts**
SECOND EDITION
Peter Harper

Obsessive Compulsive Disorder: the**facts**
THIRD EDITION
de Silva

Osteoarthritis: the**facts**
Reid et al.

Osteoporosis: the**facts**
Alison J. Black, Rena Sandison and David M. Reid

Panic Disorder: the**facts**
SECOND EDITION
Rachman

Polycystic Ovary Syndrome: the**facts**
Elsheikh and Murphy

Prostate Cancer: the**facts**
SECOND EDITION
Mason and Moffat

Psoriatic Arthritis: the**facts**
Gladman and Chandran

The Pill and other forms of hormonal
contraception: the**facts**
SIXTH EDITION
Guillebaud and MacGregor

Sleep Problems in Children and Adolescents:
the**facts**
Stores

Stroke: the**facts**
Lindley

Thyroid Disease: the**facts**
FOURTH EDITION
Thomson and Harris

Tourette Syndrome: the**facts**
SECOND EDITION
Robertson and Cavanna

thefacts

Post-traumatic stress

STEPHEN REGEL

Centre for Trauma, Resilience and Growth, Nottinghamshire Healthcare NHS Trust/University of Nottingham

STEPHEN JOSEPH

Centre for Trauma, Resilience and Growth, School of Sociology and Social Policy, University of Nottingham

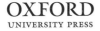

OXFORD
UNIVERSITY PRESS

OXFORD

UNIVERSITY PRESS

Great Clarendon Street, Oxford OX2 6DP

Oxford University Press is a department of the University of Oxford.
It furthers the University's objective of excellence in research, scholarship,
and education by publishing worldwide in

Oxford New York

Auckland Cape Town Dar es Salaam Hong Kong Karachi
Kuala Lumpur Madrid Melbourne Mexico City Nairobi
New Delhi Shanghai Taipei Toronto

With offices in

Argentina Austria Brazil Chile Czech Republic France Greece
Guatemala Hungary Italy Japan Poland Portugal Singapore
South Korea Switzerland Thailand Turkey Ukraine Vietnam

Oxford is a registered trade mark of Oxford University Press
in the UK and in certain other countries

Published in the United States
by Oxford University Press Inc., New York

© Oxford University Press 2010

The moral rights of the authors have been asserted
Database right Oxford University Press (maker)

First edition published 2010

British Library Cataloguing in Publication Data

Data available

Library of Congress Cataloging in Publication Data

Typeset in Plantin
by Glyph International, Bangalore, India
Printed in Great Britain on acid-free paper by Ashford Colour Press Ltd., Gosport, Hampshire

ISBN 978–0–19–956658–7

10 9 8 7 6 5 4 3 2 1

SR:

This is for Hannah and Tom for sustaining me throughout

SJ:

To Kevin and Elaine

First Foreword

Post-Traumatic Stress (PTS) and Post-Traumatic Stress Disorder (PTSD) have been given much publicity in recent years. Despite this heightened awareness, many people continue to be ignorant about PTS and PTSD, and this helpful book will certainly help explain the subject and hopefully dispel some of the myths that have grown around it.

First, it needs to be said that not everyone who passes though a traumatic incident will experience PTSD. Some individuals do experience symptoms which, if recognized and properly dealt with can enable them to resume normal life without further trouble. Others are less severely affected. It goes without saying that all experiences of severe trauma leave a mark on the individual but this mark need not be totally negative. Many people have found that although the suffering they faced was considerable, they have nevertheless been able to turn it round so that something creative, for themselves and for others, emerges from what may have appeared to be a total disaster.

The key to dealing with traumatic situations is for an expert diagnosis to be made as soon as possible after the incident. For most, this will mean relating their story before a trained listener. This alone will enable the individual to objectify their experience rather than burying it deep down inside. The very fact of 'telling the story' can be a first step in dealing constructively with the situation.

Those who view PTSD counselling with a degree of scepticism sometimes quote the terrible experiences of former Far Eastern Prisoners of War. 'They received no counselling', the argument goes, 'yet they managed perfectly well.' As one who had has a great deal to do with these men and their families, I can testify that that viewpoint is certainly not the whole truth. Many of the former prisoners on discharge were told not to talk about their experiences, but instead to 'get on with life'. In the tradition of the British 'stiff upper lip' they did so, only for many, in later life, to suffer flashbacks and nightmares, which severely disturbed their lives and the lives of their families.

One should not blame the medical authorities of the day for these troubles. In post-World War Two Britain, there was little or no knowledge of PTSD. Today, as this book reveals, there is a wealth of information available and it is being added to daily.

It is my belief that this book will help improve understanding amongst the general public, but I believe it will do more than that. It is my hope that *Post-Traumatic Stress: The Facts* will be helpful to anyone who has experienced trauma, or to those who are close to victims. It is a most valuable contribution to the growing body of literature on this subject.

Terry Waite, CBE
Chairman, Hostage UK

Foreword

Those interested in the phenomenon of post-traumatic stress have more opportunities today than ever before to learn about it. With the help of the guidance in this book sufferers may also have a greater chance to access appropriate support for dealing with their symptoms. But it was not always so.

> *'We simply needed to be reassured that our reactions*
> *were normal, that they could be recognised . . . '*

> *'Survivors often felt their families and friends had no idea how to deal with*
> *these strange people who had returned to live with them. There was no under-*
> *standing or information available at the time and no support for the families.'*

These comments by disaster survivors twenty years ago reflect the impact of trauma both on those directly affected and those around them and the fact that the kind of information included in this book was not available to them at the time when they most needed it.

It was only as recently as November 8th 2006 that responses to war-related trauma were officially addressed by the British government. Through legislation included in the 2006 Armed Forces Act, men in the British and Commonwealth armies who were executed in World War One were officially pardoned. It was not a day too soon to address the fact that so many trauma victims had been labelled as suffering from 'Soldier's Heart', 'Shell Shock', 'Combat Fatigue', 'Combat Exhaustion' or 'Operational Fatigue' because a diagnosis and treatment for PTSD had not been available to them. In 2006 the then Defence Secretary Des Browne said:

> *'I believe it is better to acknowledge that injustices were clearly done in*
> *some cases - even if we cannot say which - and to acknowledge that*
> *all these men were victims of war. I hope that pardoning these men will*
> *finally remove the stigma with which their families have lived for years.'*

It is never too late to review our understanding of the nature of trauma and society's treatment of its sufferers. This book charts the development of that understanding as well as the latest approaches to responding to such trauma.

The majority of people will experience at least one traumatic event in their lifetime and although for most this won't lead to the development of PTSD, nonetheless it is clear that information and education can make a key difference in dealing with trauma. This book can help make that difference.

Regel and Joseph offer a straightforward, understandable way of making sense of the range of reactions and responses that people may experience following traumatic events. Common questions people often have include:- *What is PTSD and how can you know if you or someone you know has it? What makes some people more likely to develop PTSD after exposure to a traumatic event than others? What helps and how can I access support? What can one expect from assessment, interventions strategies and treatment processes?* All these are addressed in this book.

It will tell you not only about the nature of traumatic experiences but how these impact on our basic assumptions about ourselves, other people, and the world in general. The authors highlight how reactions to trauma are normal responses to the kinds of circumstances sufferers have faced.

Although this is not primarily a self-help manual, it includes helpful practical tools such as questionnaires for assessing one's level of social support, and about screening for trauma. There are also helpful details about further reading and useful organizations at the end of the book.

Those of us who have encountered trauma directly and suffered from its consequences personally, socially, and politically, have come to know that having information, understanding and acknowledgement is the first step to recovery. I hope this book will assist today's sufferers, their supporters, and therapists through the wisdom of its authors and their guidance.

Dr Anne Eyre
Trauma Training and Vice-Chair, Disaster Action

Preface

The range and diversity of the human response to extremely stressful and traumatic experiences is as extensive as the different traumatic events and stressors that confront human beings. From survivors of road-traffic collisions through to those who have experienced assault and rape, war veterans, survivors of disasters both manmade and natural, and the experience of refugees, trauma cuts across all human boundaries. And now in the twenty-first century there are new threats of global catastrophy, war and terrorism. There are also the experiences of those who work in the emergency services, such as the police, fire and rescue services, health and, of course, those who work for humanitarian agencies, who have to cope with trauma and human suffering often of staggering proportions.

This little volume is aimed at providing a map of the 'landscape' of trauma and its emotional aftermath. The reader is given the necessary information, guided directions and helpful signposts in order to understand the key issues affecting the reactions of individuals, families and communities exposed to traumatic events.

We hope that this book will be helpful to people exposed to traumatic events, and to their partners, friends and families, who are themselves often in need of information. In the aftermath, confusion is common. Survivors may not understand what is happening to them. Families and friends may feel rejected and struggle to know how to help. We offer advice on some do's and don't's, as well as directions for further advice and support. For those who wish to know more, we end with suggestions, for reading and internet resources.

We have each been involved in the study, observation, research, counselling and treatment of traumatized individuals, families and communities in a variety of contexts and settings for over twenty years. Frequent requests at lectures, seminars and workshops for an accessible introduction to the range and nature of post-traumatic reactions, assessment, interventions and other aspects of the field, led us to write this book. Therefore, the secondary audience of this book is the general reader and the many professionals who come into contact with traumatized individuals—general practitioners, social workers, nurses, counsellors and psychotherapists.

This book will also be a valuable resource for those who work in high-risk professions, e.g. the emergency services, who are involved in peer support for colleagues exposed to traumatic events in the workplace and will find this an accessible introduction to the field. Over the past two decades there has also been a significant heightening of the awareness of the impact of trauma in other contexts and settings, such as in a humanitarian context, and it is hoped that this may be a useful introduction.

Finally, we owe an enormous debt of gratitude to our many clients, patients and participants in our research studies, who have taught us so much over the years and contributed to the case studies contained in many of the chapters. These are their stories, which they have generously allowed us to share, in order to illustrate and highlight many diverse experiences. They know who they are and we cannot thank them enough.

Acknowledgements

We wish to thank Liz Edwards for her patience and forbearance with her excellent administrative support. We also express our gratitude to Jenny Wright and Nic Ulyatt of Oxford University Press for their invaluable advice, patience and support throughout, and for keeping us in check and on course!

We also wish to acknowledge the contribution of many colleagues to our thinking about our work over the years. They have not only been thoughtful, caring and professional colleagues but good, 'critical' friends who have played a huge part in our continuing enthusiasm and motivation to continue with this work—thank you.

SR wishes to thank Arlene Healey from the Family Trauma Centre (FTC) in Belfast for her friendship and sound, pragmatic experience and advice over the years, as well as the excellent team at the FTC for making me feel part of the family; Dr Marion Gibson a good friend and colleague who has given me many opportunities over the years; Associate Professor Peter Berliner from the University of Copenhagen, for his warmth, enthusiasm, experience and for teaching me about 'community' approaches to trauma; Professor David Alexander, Robert Gordon University for his mentorship over the years; Dr Atle Dyregrov, Director, Centre for Crisis Psychology, Bergen for contributing so much to my thinking around early interventions for individuals, groups and families following traumatic experiences, many would do well to embrace his practical and creative approaches in the field; Dr Anne Hackmann at the Oxford Cognitive Therapy Centre for her insightful supervision; Claire Hallam at Freeth Cartwright Solicitors for helpful comments on the section on litigation. Thanks are also due in no small measure to my friend, colleague and co-author Stephen Joseph for not only keeping me on track but also to broadening and challenging my thinking about my work in trauma. Finally, there are the many colleagues and students I have come into contact with over the years

SJ would like to thank his colleagues at the University of Nottingham, particularly Professor Saul Becker, Dr Belinda Harris, David Murphy, Dr Hugh Middleton and Dr Victoria Tischler for their support over this past year; the students of the Postgraduate Certificate in Trauma Studies who have shared their experiences with me and from whom I have learned; and Steve Regel for his warmth and friendship, and whose vision it was for us to write this book. Finally, my thanks to Professor William Yule and Ruth Williams who give me my first opportunities to work in this field.

Contents

1

Common responses to traumatic events

➲ Key points

- The range of reactions following exposure to a traumatic event is wide-ranging and trauma affects different people in different ways.

- Common responses to trauma include having upsetting thoughts and images, attempting to avoid reminders, feelings of emotional numbness, being on edge and jumpy, and experiencing strong feelings of shame, guilt, anger and rage.

- When reactions become so distressing and prolonged that everyday life is affected, a person may be diagnosed as suffering from post-traumatic stress disorder (PTSD).

- Some people remain distressed for months and even years after an event, some people return to usual functioning relatively soon, and some may experience a delayed reaction to the event months or years later.

- Exposure to trauma may have a variety of other cognitive, emotional, behavioural and social consequences, such as relationship breakdown, reliance on alcohol or cigarette use as a way of coping, or impair physical health.

A brief historical introduction

Traumatic events affect different people in different ways. Most people are affected in some way when they are exposed to a traumatic event, but for most their reactions do not last long and are not too distressing. Within days or weeks most people feel as if they are back to how they were and getting on with their lives. But, for some people, reactions can be more distressing and longer lasting. As we will see in Chapter 3, there are a number of reasons for this. Some people may be less resilient at that time, perhaps due to other stressors already in their lives, and so the impact of a traumatic event affects them more significantly. For people who are affected, there is also a common core of reactions and it is these that we will first turn to. Throughout history people have recognized that traumatic events can leave people in a state of confusion, distress, and despair.

> I did within these six days see smoke still remaining of the late fire in the City; and it is strange to think how this very day I cannot sleep at night without great terrors of fire, and this very night could not sleep until almost two in the morning through thoughts of fire.

So wrote Samuel Pepys in his diary entry for the 18 February 1667, six months after the Great Fire of London in 1666. Pepys's account is perhaps one of the earliest documented descriptions of a major disaster and its aftermath. His accounts of the fire and the psychological impact it had on him provide a detailed and fascinating account of his own, and others', reactions to the effects of the fire. Physicians (the discipline of psychiatry was still in its infancy) first began to see cases in the nineteenth century of individuals exposed to industrial accidents. The industrial revolution saw the increasing mechanization of industry along with the increase of mechanized travel, e.g. the invention of the railway, which indirectly led to an early study of the impact of trauma. Herbert Page, surgeon to the London and North West Railway in 1883, used the term 'nervous shock' and described the effects of traumatic events on individuals following a rail accident thus:

> We know of no clinical picture more distressing than that of a strong and healthy man reduced by apparently inadequate causes to a state in which all control of the emotions is well-nigh gone; who cannot sleep because he has before his mind an ever-present sense of the accident; who starts at the least noise; who lies in bed almost afraid to move; whose heart palpitates whenever he is spoken to; and who cannot hear or say a word about his present condition and his future prospects without bursting into tears.

The author Charles Dickens was a passenger on a train when it crashed in Staplehurst in Kent in 1865. At the scene he witnessed many distressing sights and helped the injured and the dying. Later when safe in London, he described feeling 'quite shattered and broken up'. Some days later, clearly overwhelmed by his experience, he complained of feeling 'faint and sick' sensations in his head. In a letter to his daughter some years later, he wrote:

> I am not quite right within, but believe it to be an effect of the railway shaking.
>
> I am curiously weak—weak as if I were recovering from a long illness....

He also experienced difficulties in the years following his experience of the crash and developed a phobia of rail travel. Dickens died on the fifth anniversary of the disaster.

In the First and Second World Wars, terms like shell-shock and war neurosis were introduced to explain the presentations of soldiers affected by their combat experience. R.G. Rows, a medical physician, wrote of his experiences in the

British Medical Journal in 1916. He was treating cases of shell-shock at the Red Cross Military Hospital, Maghull and described the following reactions amongst the men he saw:

> In some cases the physical expression of a special emotion, such as fear or terror, persists for a long time without much change. This condition is usually associated with an emotional state produced by the constant intrusion of the memory of some past incident... they know they are irritable, that they are unable to interest themselves or to give a maintained attention to a given subject... all this is very real to them and leads to a condition of anxiety which is increased by their not being able to understand their condition; they worry because they fear how far this sort of thing may go.

Perhaps the earliest account of war neurosis was by the Greek historian Herodotus, who described the psychogenic (this refers to a person presenting with physical symptoms that are psychological in origin) blindness suffered by the Athenian warrior Epizelus at the battle of Marathon in 490 BC:

> Epizelus, the son of Cuphagorus, an Athenian soldier, was fighting bravely when he suddenly lost the sight of both eyes, though nothing had touched him anywhere—neither sword, spear, nor missile. From that moment he continued blinded as long as he lived. I am told that in speaking about what happened to him he used to say that he fancied he was opposed by a man of great stature in heavy armour, whose beard overshadowed his shield, but the phantom passed him by and killed the man at his side.

Common reactions to traumatic events

Much of the time our lives seem safe and predictable. Serious road-traffic collisions, plane crashes, train accidents, natural disasters, criminal assaults and other sorts of traumatic events seem to happen to other people, not us. We may read about them in the papers, or watch them on TV, but we do not expect to experience them directly ourselves.

But for those of us who have gone through trauma, we know that any of us, at any time, can be the victims of sudden and unexpected tragedies or losses. Sadly, things can, and sometimes do, happen to us or to people we are close to, and not just to other people in other places. If they do, we are likely to experience a range of unfamiliar feelings and reactions associated with the shock of the event and may have some difficulty in collecting our thoughts and handling our feelings about what has happened.

There are no 'right' or 'wrong' ways to react, and different people exposed to the same trauma may respond in quite different ways. Although everyone's experience will be unique and personal, the process of psychological adjustment and recovery will often be different.

While most people involved in a traumatic incident will be shaken by what has happened, some adjust to their experiences with little or no apparent distress and emerge emotionally unscathed. This would be considered a quite common response. Sometimes people may in fact feel satisfied by the way that they have acted when faced by the traumatic event (e.g. if they have been able to help others who have been involved).

Other people, however, are shocked and stunned by the traumatic event, and have difficulty believing what has happened to them. In the days following the incident, some people feel confused, distressed and fearful, or experience other emotions or reactions, which can in themselves be unpleasant and worrying. Even though such reactions can seem strange, it is important to understand (and explain) that they are also entirely normal and understandable responses to severe stress and shock. In most cases the reactions, are short-lived and pass after a few days or weeks.

Below are some common feelings, emotions and behaviours sometimes experienced or displayed by survivors (and sometimes also by witnesses, relatives and emergency workers), in the hours, days and some weeks following an extremely stressful or traumatic event. These can include any of the following.

Psychological reactions

- Anxiety—feelings of fearfulness, nervousness or sometimes panic, especially when faced by reminders of the event; concerns about losing control or not coping; worry that the situation may recur.

- Hyper-vigilance—constantly scanning the environment for cues of danger or seeing threat in things that would have appeared innocent before. This could mean being overly protective of children or loved ones, e.g. worrying if they are slightly late home or haven't phoned at exactly the time they said they would.

- Sleep disturbance—difficulty in getting off to sleep, restless sleep, vivid dreams or nightmares. At first these may be about the incident itself or the experience, but they can change to be less specific, where the content can just be unsettling or generally disturbing.

- Intrusive memories—intrusive thoughts/images of the traumatic incident, which can appear to 'come out of the blue', without any triggers or reminders. Other thoughts, images or feelings may be prompted by media triggers, e.g. something on TV, newspapers, sounds, a song or piece of music, smells.

- Guilt—feelings of regret, about not having acted or coped as well as one would have wished, about letting one's self or others down, about being in some way responsible. Other feelings of guilt may be present because the person survived, whilst a friend or loved one died—again, this is a common phenomenon and is known as 'survivor guilt'. Often when we feel guilt we want to make things right again somehow.

- Shame or embarrassment—feelings related to how we think of ourselves, often related to a sense that we were not good enough in some way. When we feel shame we want to go into hiding.

- Sadness—feelings of low mood and tearfulness.

- Irritability and anger—at what happened, the injustice of the event; 'Why me?' at those you feel are responsible for the trauma and wanting somebody to accept responsibility or blame. Irritability can often be directed at loved ones, close family, friends or colleagues.

- Emotional numbness or blunting—feeling detached from others or being unable to experience emotions such love or happiness.

- Withdrawal—tending to retreat into one's self, avoiding social and family contact.

- Disappointment—thinking that people (including family) do not really understand how you are feeling.

- Mental avoidance—avoiding thoughts to do with the trauma. People try to push distressing thoughts out of their head, often unsuccessfully, and in the longer term this can cause further problems because it interferes with the person processing and making sense of their experience.

- Behavioural avoidance—avoiding thoughts, feelings, activities that are reminders of the trauma. These can be often subtle at first, such as avoiding noisy or crowded environments, taking a different route to work and so on. There is also the potential for these avoidances and fears to spread or 'generalize' to other situations; in other words, to experience similar sensations when in situations that have a semblance or resonance to the original trauma. This may mean that someone who feels anxious and avoids driving after a car accident, may start to feel anxious and avoid travelling by other forms of transport, e.g. by bus, train or develop a fear of flying. Again Dickens, two years after his accident, in 1867, described having 'sudden, vague rushes of terror, even when riding in a hansom cab, which are perfectly unreasonable but quite insurmountable...'.

- An increased startle response—becoming 'jumpy' or easily startled by sudden noises or movements, e.g. a door slamming shut, the phone or door bell ringing.

Physical reactions

The person may also have certain bodily sensations, with or without the psychological reactions described above. Many of these symptoms are signs of anxiety, tension, or stress. For example:

- Shakiness and trembling.
- Tension and muscular aches (especially in the head and neck).
- Insomnia, tiredness, fatigue.

- Poor concentration, forgetfulness.
- Palpitations, shallow rapid breathing, dizziness.
- Gastrointestinal symptoms such as nausea, vomiting and diarrhoea.
- Disturbance of menstrual cycle or loss of interest in sex.

Impact on relationships

As we will see in Chapter 8 (Growth following adversity), in some cases a shared sense of adversity or loss can bring people closer together, help create new bonds or strengthen relationships. But although family and friends are usually understanding and supportive, the experience of trauma can sometimes also place strains on relationships. The person may feel that too little, or the wrong sort of help and support is offered, or that others do not appreciate what they have been through and expect too much of them. Sometimes, when relationships become strained, there is a tendency for people to rely on alcohol or drugs as a means of coping. For others, such as Laura, there may be thoughts of suicide.

Laura's story

Laura is an experienced mental health nurse who was present when a female patient walked into the day unit she was working in and poured a can of petrol over herself and then set fire to herself. The patient ran into a toilet and locked herself in. She tried for several minutes to save the woman who was on fire and, despite many attempts, failed to reach her and prevent her from burning to death. At first Laura felt that she had coped well with a very traumatic experience and that her experience and training would assist in that coping. However, in the weeks that followed, she found she was experiencing a range of reactions that were becoming more intense and increasing in frequency, intensity and duration. Her irritability was increasing, especially towards her partner. She was having difficulty concentrating, sleeping, having anxiety and panic attacks and felt as though 'she was losing it'. This was most characterized by her extreme reaction one day. 'I was in my bedroom trashing the place and feeling as though I wanted to hurt myself...'. Reflecting on her experiences she recalled, '...the day after the incident I was offered counselling. I thought "Why would I need counselling?". Why didn't anyone think to explain how we might feel and what we needed to look out for... the last six months have been absolutely awful... I never thought I would feel suicidal or want to abandon my partner of 10 years'.

As was noted by Rows with soldiers from the First World War, the phrase '...this is very real to them and leads to a condition of anxiety which is increased by their not being able to understand their condition...' has a resonance with many individuals we have seen who have been exposed to traumatic events.

They often do not know what is happening to them or what is common or normal for them in their particular circumstances, something evidenced above in Laura's story.

It is again important to emphasize that there are no right or wrong ways to react after a traumatic experience or bereavement. Everyone's reactions will be individual and not everybody will experience all of the feelings described above, nor experience them to the same degree.

Reactions will vary from person to person for a number of reasons, including:

◆ Differences in personality.

◆ Ways of expressing emotion.

◆ Styles and methods of coping.

◆ Previous experiences of adversity or trauma.

◆ The extent to which there are existing stresses and strains in other areas of their lives.

◆ The exact nature of the traumatic event and the individual or families experience will also make a difference.

◆ If the incident was violent, extraordinary and unexpected.

◆ Witnessing death and serious injuries.

◆ If the individual was seriously injured, this can also affect subsequent reactions, by numbing or delaying the psychological impact.

While most people will have at least short-lived feelings of shakiness, jumpiness, anxiety or anger, some will have none or milder reactions, dependent on the factors mentioned above, including their proximity to the event. However, in the immediate aftermath and following days, the person has intense or unpleasant physical reactions, sleep disturbance, intrusive memories, feelings of fear or guilt, or other reactions of the type described above, it cannot be over-emphasized that these are entirely common and normal reactions to abnormal events and in most cases are not long-lasting.

Post-traumatic stress disorder (PTSD)

Whilst it has been noticed that there was a common core to how people react, for some, those whose reactions become more intense, frequent, upsetting and begin to interfere with everyday life, this can often be the manifestation of what is now known as post-traumatic stress disorder or PTSD.

PTSD reactions are grouped into three sections:

1. Re-experiencing of the traumatic event.

2. Numbing of responsiveness to, or reduced involvement in, the external world.

3. A miscellaneous section, which includes memory impairment, difficulty concentrating, hyper-alertness or an exaggerated startle response.

What is PTSD?

- PTSD is the term used by psychiatrists to describe reactions that cause clinically significant distress or impairment in social, occupational or other important areas of functioning in people who have experienced a traumatic event.

- A traumatic event is defined in this case as an event that involves actual or threatened death or serious injury, or a threat to the physical health of self or others, and in which the person felt frightened, horrified and helpless.

- When people experience traumatic events they may have distressing recollections including images, thought, and distressing dreams. It may even be that it seems as if the event were happening again.

- When there are reminders, the person may experience distress and feel shaken up. As a result, people often try to avoid reminders, such as thoughts, feelings, conversations associated with the trauma, or activities, places or people that bring back memories.

- People may also shut down mentally and emotionally and have trouble remembering what happened, feel cut off from others and have difficulty in having loving feelings. There may also be difficulties falling or staying asleep, irritability or outbursts of anger and difficulty concentrating.

- When the above problems last for more than a month, then a diagnosis of PTSD can be made. A full description of the diagnostic criteria for PTSD is provided by the National Centre for PTSD (see: http://ncptsd. kattare.com/ncmain/ncdocs/fact_shts/fs_dsm_iv_tr.html).

Who is most at risk?

No one knows in advance how anyone may react to a particular stressful event. All the same, what happens after extreme stress is to some extent dependent on what was happening in the person's life before the event, what they did during the event, how they dealt with the demands of the situation and some immediate or early reactions they may have had to their experience.

For instance, if life prior to the event had been troubled through difficulties within their family, feeling alone, unexpected changes or upheavals, loss or bereavements or poor health, reactions may be more marked than had circumstances been more favourable. Factors affecting risk and vulnerability, as well as factors that impact on the individual's recovery, will be covered in more detail in Chapter 4. PTSD cannot be diagnosed until at least one month has passed since the trauma. This is to recognize that, in the early days, it is common for people to experience these reactions and it is only when they become persistent that mental health professionals need to really take notice.

Acute stress disorder

In the first month if people are experiencing problems, psychiatrists talk about acute stress disorder. This is like PTSD but, because PTSD cannot be diagnosed until a month has passed, this recognizes that people can still be affected. After a month, if the person is still affected, the person would then be said to have PTSD.

What is trauma?

In both acute stress disorder and PTSD, the first thing is the description of what is a trauma:

◆ exposure to a traumatic event;

◆ the person's reaction or response to it.

It is important to recognize that people must experience a traumatic event for diagnoses of either acute stress disorder or PTSD, but everyone reacts differently—so what is traumatic for one person may not be traumatic for another. It is important to understand each person's reactions, and what the trauma means to them.

World Health Organization

Both acute stress disorder and PTSD were developed by the American Psychiatric Association and the above descriptions are the ones that are most commonly used in the Western world. But it should be noted that the World Health Organization (WHO) also includes within its most recent edition of the International Classification of Diseases three diagnoses:

1. Acute stress disorder.

2. Post-traumatic stress disorder.

3. Adjustment disorder.

Acute stress disorder describes a condition that develops in an individual following exposure to a traumatic event. Reactions often may appear, usually within minutes or hours of the event, and often subside but are expected to last no longer than 2–3 days at the most. There may be an initial state of 'daze'; disorientation, panic, anxiety, are commonly present. However, some studies have shown that if this occurs and is sustained over a period of more than a week or so within the first month, then it may be a predictor of later PTSD.

PTSD includes re-experiencing the event, or what are often described as 'flashbacks'. It must be noted here that real 'flashbacks' are often accompanied by a sensory modality, such as touch, taste or smell, and the individual feels that they are actually re-experiencing the event as if it were happening again, e.g. they *feel* as though they are back in the burning car, or can *actually smell* the body odour of their assailant. In addition, they may lose a conscious awareness of their surroundings for a few moments or minutes, as illustrated by the following quote from a woman who survived a rail crash:

> I suddenly experience a whooshing sound and feel as if I'm back in the carriage.

They may experience dreams, which occur against the persisting background of a sense of 'numbness' and emotional blunting, detachment from other people, unresponsiveness and avoidance of activities and situations reminiscent of the trauma. Commonly, there is fear and avoidance of cues that remind the sufferer of the original trauma. Rarely, there may be dramatic, acute bursts of fear, panic or aggression, triggered by stimuli arousing a sudden recollection and/or re-enactment of the trauma or of the original reaction to it, an enhanced startle reaction, and insomnia. Anxiety and depression are commonly associated with the above symptoms and signs, and suicidal ideation may be present. Excessive use of alcohol or drugs may also be a complicating factor.

Adjustment disorders refer to states of subjective and emotional disturbance that arise in the period of adaptation to a significant life change or to the consequences of a stressful event, affecting the person's social network through, for example, bereavement. Although it is assumed that the condition would not have arisen without the stressor, what differentiates this category from that of PTSD is the acknowledgement of the role of individual differences. Symptoms are thought to include depressed mood, anxiety, worry, a feeling of inability to cope, to plan ahead or to continue in the present situation, and some degree of disability in the performance of daily routine.

The effects of trauma can be very long-lasting. Studies have shown survivors of disaster and other extreme events, such as sexual assault, remain affected many years later.

Indeed, PTSD has even been shown in World War II veterans and survivors of the Holocaust fifty years later. But although problems can exist many years later, people may not be continuously troubled all of that time. A number of people do not develop problems initially, but only months or even years later.

Other reactions

The diagnosis of PTSD represents a core of reactions experienced by survivors of traumatic events; but trauma affects different people differently. As well as these core reactions, people's personality can be affected, sometimes referred to as 'post-traumatic character disorder'.

Many people also report high levels of both anxiety and depression. Negative emotional states (e.g. rage, anger, guilt, shame) are common (see Box below). As well as guilt and shame, there may be intense feelings of rage and anger. Such negative emotional states are distressing and can lead to destructive behaviours, such as substance abuse, in an attempt to dull or block them. Substance use in survivors of traumatic events is also common.

Survivors of the *Herald of Free Enterprise*

In 1987, a passenger cruise ship, the *Herald of Free Enterprise*, left harbour in Zeebrugge *en route* to Dover. But, a few minutes out of harbour, water started pouring in through the bow doors, which had not been properly secured. Passengers and crew, oblivious to the danger, were ordering food in the restaurants, and settling in to their journey. Without warning, the ship began to lurch and, in less than a minute, had capsized. 193 people died that day in one of the most horrific maritime disasters of the twentieth century.

A group of psychologists contacted survivors three years later and asked them to take part in a survey. It was found that:

◆ over half felt guilt for being alive when so many died;

◆ approximately a third said that they felt guilty about things they did;

◆ two-thirds said that they felt guilty about things they failed to do;

◆ almost a third said that they felt they had let themselves down during the disaster;

◆ almost half said that they felt they had let others down.

In survivors of the Herald of Free Enterprise it was also found that:

◆ 73% reported that their alcohol consumption had increased;

◆ 44% reported that their cigarette consumption had increased;

◆ 40% reported that their use of sleeping tablets had increased;

◆ 28% reported that their use of anti-depressants had increased;

◆ 21% reported that their use of tranquillisers had increased.

There may also be physical health problems, including tiredness, headaches, chest pains, gastrointestinal disorders, cardiovascular disorders, renal disorders, respiratory diseases and infectious diseases, as well as impairments in the immune system. Trauma may also affect social relationships because of increased levels of irritability, withdrawal and decreased enjoyment from shared activities, leading to marital and interfamilial discord, and sometimes even domestic violence.

2

Concepts and theories
of post-traumatic stress

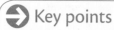 **Key points**

◆ Theories provide us with a pair of spectacles through which to look at our own or other peoples' reactions to trauma.

◆ Psychologists, psychiatrists and counsellors use theory to plan therapy.

◆ Biological, behavioural, psychodynamic, social-cognitive and integrative theories are reviewed.

Introduction

In this chapter we will discuss the theories of trauma. Much theoretical work has been carried out in the field of psychological trauma, since PTSD was first introduced. A variety of theories of psychological trauma have been put forward.

We will examine the main theoretical perspectives that have been presented for understanding trauma. Firstly, we will review the biological perspective. Secondly, we will look at the concept of emotional processing as proposed by Rachman. Third, the psychodynamically informed information-processing approach of Horowitz. Fourth, the social cognitive ideas surrounding 'shattered assumptions' put forward by Janoff-Bulman. We will then examine the dual representation theory proposed by Brewin and colleagues, and the cognitive model of PTSD as developed by Ehlers and Clark. Finally, we will discuss the integrative psychosocial approach of Joseph, Williams and Yule.

The aim is to provide the reader with a sketch of the different theoretical perspectives. Although it is beyond the scope of the present book to provide a comprehensive examination of each perspective, the reader will be equipped with knowledge that will be useful to them in making sense of their own or other peoples' reactions, and in talking things through with health professionals.

Biological perspective

A good starting point is the recognition that post-traumatic stress reactions, such as being on a state of constant alertness, having an excessive startle response, focused concentration, are characteristic of a special 'survival mode' of functioning. A key feature of PTSD is that individuals continue to experience fear and danger in the absence of any real danger given that the original threat has passed. This of course is very different to experiencing fear and other symptoms where threat and danger is ever present, such as in situations where there is ongoing civil conflict, persistent threat as in domestic violence, and other similar situations. In situations where there is continuous traumatic stress, then states of constant alertness, having an excessive startle response and so on, make sense as the person is prepared to react in survival mode. In essence, the biological perspective is that PTSD is caused by the biological mechanisms that are activated during trauma, and which are adaptive during trauma, but somehow fail to switch off once the danger is past. So the person remains in survival mode.

From a biological perspective it could be seen that individuals who display marked symptoms of post-traumatic stress have been biologically primed to respond to danger where none exists. The emotion of fear is a normal and characteristic emotional response to threat and danger and this in turn is influenced by our memory of what represents threatening situations or what they have meant in specific instances in experience and in our past.

Usually there three types of responses known to us all: flight, fight or freeze. The last of these may serve a protective purpose and occasionally when individuals are faced with significant threat a phenomenon known as dissociation, which may occur around the time of the traumatic event and can lead to a variety of sensations, such as the person thinking that time has slowed down, things are moving in slow motion and they may lose awareness of their surroundings. Parts of the brain are thought to be activated when individuals are exposed to traumatic situations to allow the flight or fight or freeze mechanisms to be activated and that means that some people are not able to 'switch off'. Such reactions are likely to be adaptive as they enable people to respond to dangerous situations, thus increasing the chance of survival. From an evolutionary perspective, post-traumatic reactions might be adaptive in many situations and might therefore be considered to be a normal and adaptive reaction. A similar evolutionary significance might be attached to the protective function of dissociation when stress exceeds coping resources' capacity. However, it is the persistence of reactions and their interference with everyday social functioning that is a problem.

The work of Pierre Janet

These ideas can be traced back to Pierre Janet (1859–1947) who originally embarked upon his professional career as a professor of philosophy but later became interested in the phenomena of hypnosis and rose to great prominence in international psychiatry during the turn of the twentieth century. Despite dying in virtual obscurity, and many of his ideas being swept away by Freud's teachings, which became the principal psychological theory of much of the twentieth century, Janet is now seen as one of the seminal thinkers and contributors to our understanding of the impact of trauma on individuals. Janet thought that people exposed to traumatic events suffered from a loss of capacity to store and utilize conscious information.

Janet suggested that intense emotional reactions cause memories of particular events to be dissociated from consciousness and to be stored as visceral sensations (panic and anxiety) or visual images (nightmares and flashbacks). These intense emotions interfere with the integration of the experience into existing memory schemas. Janet (1909) considered dissociation, in the context of trauma, to result from a state of physiological hyper-arousal, which results in memory disturbance. Dissociation can be described as a range of processes that involve 'the destruction of the usually integrated feelings of consciousness, memory, identity and perception of the environment' (examples of dissociation will be given in Chapter 4). The information conveyed by the traumatic event is not available to ordinary conscious representation and so cannot be processed. Instead it persists as a fixed idea that is split off from consciousness and experienced in nightmares.

Janet wrote in 1930:

> I was forced to recognise in certain cases the role of one or several events in a person's past experience. These events, which had precipitated a violent emotion and a destruction of the psychological system had left traces. The memory of these events and the mental energy involved in keeping them at bay absorbed a great deal of energy, leading to continuing deterioration.

Janet believed that the initial emotional reaction to the traumatic event (which he referred to as 'vehement emotion') dictated the intensity of post-traumatic reactions. He believed that when people get very upset they stop being able to make sense of an experience and can no longer work out what action to take to escape. Modern studies have supported Janet's belief that post-traumatic reactions originate in 'vehement emotions' that are biologically encoded. Contemporary research also supports the idea that the initial level of physical arousal predicts the severity of the response. For example, in a study that followed survivors of an oil-rig disaster in the North Sea of Scotland, it was found that the severity of dissociative symptoms predicted longer term distress.

Rachman's emotional processing theory

Turning now to the behavioural perspective, one idea that we find very useful is 'emotional processing'. This is an idea introduced by a psychologist called Stanley Rachman in 1980 before the term PTSD was formally introduced.

What Rachman did was to observe that many different emotional and behavioural reactions experienced by people, such as grief, nightmares, obsessions, could all be understood as manifestations of a failure to emotionally process an upsetting experience. The concept of emotional processing, therefore, provides a powerful theoretical perspective with which to understand a diversity of seemingly unrelated phenomena. Thus, when the concept of PTSD was introduced, with its hallmark symptoms of re-experiencing, avoidance and hyper-arousal, Rachman's theory allowed us to conceptualize PTSD as indicative of incomplete emotional processing.

Rachman's theory suggested was that we have a need to absorb emotional reactions. So, following a trauma there may be a lot of emotional confusion and distress, but over time most people are able to absorb their emotional reactions. However, not everyone does so and that's when we see post-traumatic stress reactions, such as upsetting dreams, nightmares and so on. Rachman (1980) writes:

> Broadly, successful processing can be gauged from the person's ability to talk about, see, listen to or be reminded of the emotional events without experiencing distress or disruptions.

He proposed various factors, which give rise to difficulties in emotional processing. Events that are sudden, intense, dangerous, uncontrollable and unpredictable are harder to absorb emotionally. People with a more anxious personality, who are in a state of fatigue, who have other stressors in their lives and who have problems expressing themselves, will have difficulties emotionally processing or making sense of extremely stressful events.

The emotional processing theory of Rachman can help us understand how people are able to return to pre-trauma states. In summary, his approach provided three important perspectives. First, a conceptual framework within which to understand a range of previously disparate phenomena. Second, that people have some form of intrinsically motivated drive toward processing powerful new emotional information. Third, that processing itself could be promoted or impeded by various events, personality, activity and emotional states.

Horowitz's information-processing theory

Moving to thinking derived from the psychodynamic perspective, Mardi Horowitz provides what we think is another useful way of understanding trauma. Horowitz's approach is based on the idea that people have mental models, or beliefs, about the world and of themselves, which they use to interpret their experiences. He also proposes that there is an inherent drive to make our mental models coherent with current information (what he called the 'completion principle'). In this respect, Horowitz's theory is similar to that of Rachman in proposing that people have some innate need to 'work through' or process emotional experience.

Horowitz says that a traumatic event presents information that is incompatible with existing beliefs. This incongruity gives rise to a stress response requiring reappraisal and revision of the schema. As traumatic events generally require massive changes in worldview, complete integration and cognitive processing take some time to occur. During this time, active memory tends to repeat its representations of the traumatic event, causing emotional distress; this manifests itself as the intrusive re-experiencing of the event. Re-experiencing symptoms mean that the person is in the process of working through, but this is distressing and therefore prolonged re-experiencing can be too much for the person so they move into an avoidant phase to prevent emotional exhaustion.

Thus, there is a process of inhibition and facilitation, which acts as a feedback system modulating the flow of information. The symptoms observed during stress responses, which Horowitz categorizes as involving denials and intrusion, occur as a result of opposite actions of a control system that regulates the incoming information to tolerable doses. If inhibitory control is not strong enough, intrusive symptoms, such as nightmares and flashbacks, emerge. When inhibitory efforts are too strong in relation to active memory, symptoms indicative of the avoidance phase occur (see Figure 2.1).

Typically, avoidance and intrusion symptoms fluctuate in a way particular to the individual without causing flooding or exhaustion that would prevent adaptation. The person oscillates between the states of avoidance and intrusion until a relative equilibrium is reached when the person is said to have worked through the experience. The emotional numbing symptoms are thus viewed as a defence mechanism against intrusion. Horowitz suggests that there are phases of intrusion and avoidance as the person gradually doses themselves with information.

So, intrusive and avoidant states characteristic of post-traumatic reactions are to be expected in the aftermath of a traumatic event, as the person emotionally

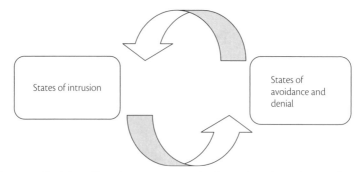

States of intrusion

States of avoidance and denial

Figure 2.1 Denials and intrusion occur as a result of opposite actions of a control system.

processers their experiences. But, not everyone successfully works through their experience and for some the process can get stuck. While intrusive memories are a universal phenomenon indicative of a normal process of working through, over time, if emotional processing is unsatisfactory, then persistent memories represent the failure of emotional processing. The longer the time elapsed since the trauma, the more likely intrusive thoughts will predict poor outcome.

In summary, the information-processing approach of Horowitz draws our attention to the central role that memory plays in the development of post-traumatic stress reactions. It is the completion tendency that maintains the trauma-related information in what Horowitz refers to as active memory, causing it to intrude into consciousness in the forms of flashbacks, nightmares and unwanted thoughts, as the individual endeavours to merge the new information with pre-existing models of the self and the world. In essence, the completion tendency serves as the driver for processing to take place. Such an approach is, therefore, compatible with Rachman's concept of emotional processing: Both emphasize that post-traumatic stress reactions are signs of incomplete processing, and point toward an intrinsic need to absorb and integrate trauma-related information regarding the event.

Janoff-Bulman's social cognitive approach

Janoff-Bulman's social cognitive approach suggests that there are common psychological experiences shared by victims who have experienced a wide range of traumatic situations. She proposed that post-traumatic stress following victimization is largely due to the disruption of three core assumptions about, the world, self and others: (1) the world as benevolent; (2) the world as meaningful; and (3) the self as worthy. Coping with victimization involves the person coming to terms with these shattered assumptions and re-establishing a conceptual system that will allow them to function effectively. Janoff-Bulman (1992) proposes that there is extensive mental rumination and processing as the person attempts to make sense of their experience and to re-establish their world-view. She distinguishes between automatic processes and intentional efforts to restructure what she described as our assumptive world.

Similarly, Epstein (1991) referred to trauma as the 'atom smasher' of personality. He proposed the cognitive-experiential self-theory, which distinguishes between two ways in which people apprehend reality, and organize experience: one intuitive, narrative, and experiential; the other analytic, deliberate and rational. These two systems, the experiential and the rational, are reciprocally influential, but it is the experiential system that is dominant and that is threatened by the experience of adversity. Drawing on Horowitz's theory, Janoff-Bulman's approach accommodates the notion of the completion tendency, and that people are intrinsically motivated to make sense of and find meaning in their experiences.

Dual representation theory

Of course, these processes take place out of conscious awareness. Emotional processing involves both 'verbally accessible memories' (VAMS) that we can deliberately retrieve from our store of autobiographical experiences and consists of 'situationally accessible memories' (SAMs). SAMs contain information that cannot be deliberately accessed by the individual and are not available for editing. Therefore, SAMs, as the name suggests, are accessed only when aspects of the original traumatic situation cue their activation, e.g. a sight, sound or smell. These represented within a completely personal context and they contain sensory information, e.g. taste, smell and other information concerning personal meanings about the traumatic event. VAMs are characterized by their ability to be deliberately retrieved and edited by a traumatized individual. It is argued that VAM representations contain the sensory, response and meaning information about the traumatic event.

This theory proposes that VAM and SAM representations are encoded in parallel at the time of the trauma, and between them they account for the range of PTSD symptoms. Brewin and colleagues (1996) proposed that individuals need to consciously integrate the verbally accessible information in VAM with their pre-existing beliefs and models of the world, and thereby restore a sense of safety and control through making appropriate adjustments to expectations about their self and the world.

Cognitive model of PTSD

Ehlers and Clark (2000) developed a cognitive model of PTSD. They propose that persistent PTSD only develops if an individual processes the trauma in a way that causes them to experience a sense of ongoing current threat. This threat might result from re-living symptoms (e.g. flashbacks), the impact the trauma has had on their perception of the world (e.g. the world is not a safe place), negative appraisals of the self during the trauma (e.g. I could have prevented this) or negative appraisals of the self post-trauma (e.g. I'm a useless person because I am not coping). The emotion that most readily corresponds with the notion of threat in PTSD is fear; however, the model proposed by Ehlers and Clark allows attention to be paid to other emotions and the role these might play in the development of ongoing current threat. They suggest that current ongoing threat can be seen as external, such as seeing the world as a more dangerous place (fear), or internal, such as seeing oneself as a less capable or acceptable human being. Such appraisals can generate strong emotions: one that is particularly relevant is the emotion of shame. It has been proposed that shame can act as an internal current threat by attacking the individual's psychological integrity leaving them feeling inferior, socially unattractive and powerless, thereby maintaining their PTSD symptoms.

Psychosocial approach

In Joseph, William and Yule's psychosocial framework, it is proposed that traumatic events present people with information that, as perceived *at the time*, gives rise to extreme emotional arousal. Representations of these *event stimuli* are held in memory, due to their personal salience and to the difficulty they present for immediate emotional processing. These *event cognitions* will idiosyncratically reflect the individual's personality and their environment and social context.

Event cognitions can then form the subject of further cognitive activity called *appraisals*. Appraisal cognitions are distinguished from traumatic cognitions in being thoughts about the information depicted and its further meanings. How one appraises an event is influenced by personality, emotional state and *coping*. Any stimulus is capable of being perceived in a variety of ways: what is dangerous to an inhabitant of Manhattan may not seem so to someone who has lived on the Ganges and vice versa.

Appraisal processes lead to various *emotional states* (e.g. fear, panic, grief, guilt and shame). The occurrence of these event appraisals and emotional states will all engender attempts at coping, which may either be active problem-solving strategies or avoidant thoughts and behaviours.

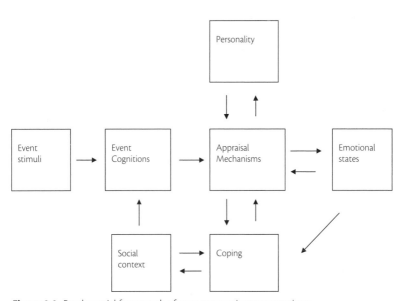

Figure 2.2 Psychosocial framework of post-traumatic stress reactions.

In this model, which is schematically represented in Figure 2.2, individual variation is attributable to a complex interaction between components that constitute variables that may contribute to outcomes at different points in time.

Using theory to plan for change

Theory helps clinicians think about the problems that people experience following trauma and how to help. To illustrate, John was in a car accident in which his fiancée died. Although it was not John's fault, he blames himself for what had happened. This reflects John's personality, which is more pessimistic than optimistic. As a result he feels ashamed and guilty. As a result of these feelings, John tries to avoid thinking about what happened and avoids other people who he feels will judge him. Over time he becomes socially isolated, in part because of his own avoidance, and in part because other people don't know how to react and withdraw from John to minimize their own discomfort (see Figure 2.3). Over time this becomes a self-perpetuating cycle of appraisals, emotional states and coping, in which John becomes mired down in shame and guilt, socially withdrawn and increasingly depressed, with thoughts of taking his own life.

John is referred to the psychologist who helps him understand his cycle of appraisals, emotional states and coping, and how, over time, they fed into each other and led to a downward spiral into depression. Together they discussed ways in

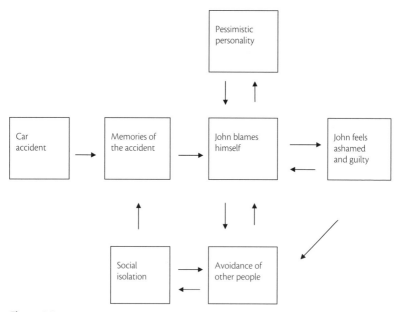

Figure 2.3

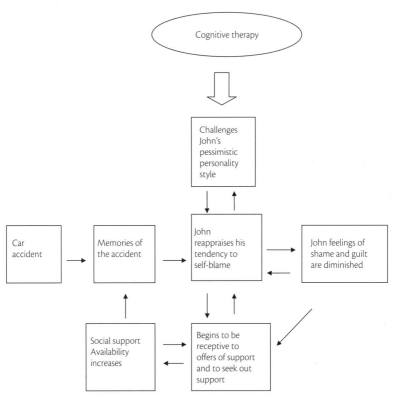

Figure 2.4

which John could change in order to put the cycle into reverse. A programme was developed involving cognitive therapy in order to challenge John's pessimistic thinking, in order to build his personal resources to deal with his negative appraisals, alongside a behavioural intervention to teach John new skills in coping and seeking support (see Figure 2.4). Over time, as John practices his new skills, he is able to increase his social support and challenge his negative thinking.

Conclusions

Theories offer us a pair of spectacles through which to look at psychological trauma. Each theory offers us something different. Theory is useful, and therapists will use theory to make sense of what their clients' tell them and to plan interventions.

3

Assessment and formulation

⮞ Key points

- The majority of people will experience at least one traumatic event in their life time.

- Most people are affected in some way by trauma but are quickly able to return to their normal state, while some people develop severe and long-lasting problems.

- PTSD can occur at any age, including childhood.

- Men tend to experience more traumatic events than women, but women often tend to experience higher impact of events.

- Women are more likely to develop PTSD in response to traumatic events than men.

The prevalence of trauma reactions and PTSD in the community

How common is PTSD? The life-time prevalence of developing PTSD following exposure to traumatic events has been estimated by research to be approximately 10.4% for women and 5% for men. There may be a number of reasons for this. For example, men and women may experience different types of traumatic events. And they may have different ways of coping.

Furthermore, different types of traumatic events are associated with different rates of PTSD. For example, rape has been associated with the highest PTSD rates in a number of research studies, as have childhood neglect, physical and sexual abuse, physical attack, being threatened, kidnapped or being held hostage. Again a number of studies tend to show different prevalence rates across different populations exposed to trauma and accidents.

Most people do not go on to develop serious and long-lasting problems. Individuals, families and communities can often cope effectively following exposure to traumatic events by utilizing their own resources. Whilst this may often be true, as indicated by the quote below, there are some people who may be vulnerable for reasons outlined later.

> What we've lost in the PTSD discourse is what they knew in the Second World War, par excellence... which is that people's reaction to trauma, adversity, war and terror is determined by the group psychology and not individual psychology. Now we're beginning to remind ourselves that normal people are pretty resilient. They have their own resources; they can maximise their social support...... People are usually the best judges of what they need, and when.

Professor Simon Wessely, 'After Shock',
The Guardian Weekend, 17 June 2006

The most important factor is social support from our community, friends, families, workplace colleagues and so on. When we have strong social support, we are most able to buffer what life throws at us. It may be worth completing the brief questionnaire in Figure 3.1 to assess your levels of social support.

To calculate your score, add up questions 1 to 5. If you scored over 25 this would indicate that you have a high degree of social support. If you scored under 25, it may be that your support could be strengthened in some ways. Other people can also say or do things that upset us or don't seem helpful in other ways. Look at your answer to question 6. Take some time to think about the things that other people do and how you would like things to be different. There is also an acknowledgement amongst many mental health professionals that not everyone has access to good social support for a variety of reasons. Furthermore, the nature and constituency of communities are changing, with social isolation becoming an increasing feature of urban and rural life.

One thing that is well-known from all the research on trauma and post-traumatic responses is that not everyone who is exposed to a traumatic event goes on to develop PTSD or other problems, which have been described previously, such as anxiety, depression and other psychiatric conditions. Therefore, why is it that some people are more likely to develop problems than others? Other findings from the research on PTSD in the community indicate that people at risk of developing post-traumatic reactions include:

- ◆ Exposed to/or have witnessed extreme traumatic events, such as physical and sexual abuse, natural or man-made disasters, road-traffic collisions, serious crime or military action.

- ◆ Those considered as special 'at-risk' populations, such as emergency service workers, e.g. the police and ambulance personnel, are often more likely to have an increased risk of exposure and could therefore be seen to be more at risk of developing post-traumatic reactions. Therefore, occupational health and welfare departments in the emergency services need to pay close attention to the welfare of such groups (see Chapter 4).

Support in a time of crisis

We are interested in the help that you received from family and friends following the event you described. Please answer the questions that follow by circling the appropriate number from the scale below:

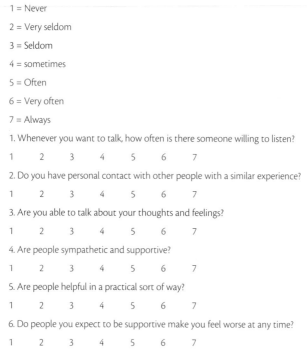

1 = Never

2 = Very seldom

3 = Seldom

4 = sometimes

5 = Often

6 = Very often

7 = Always

1. Whenever you want to talk, how often is there someone willing to listen?

1   2   3   4   5   6   7

2. Do you have personal contact with other people with a similar experience?

1   2   3   4   5   6   7

3. Are you able to talk about your thoughts and feelings?

1   2   3   4   5   6   7

4. Are people sympathetic and supportive?

1   2   3   4   5   6   7

5. Are people helpful in a practical sort of way?

1   2   3   4   5   6   7

6. Do people you expect to be supportive make you feel worse at any time?

1   2   3   4   5   6   7

Figure 3.1 Questionnaire for assessing levels of social support. Joseph, S., Andrews, B., Williams, R., & Yale, W. (1992). Reproduced with permission from the *British Journal of Clinical Psychology*, **31**, 63–73. © The British Psychological Society.

♦ Many refugees and asylum seekers have also experienced a range of traumatic events, such as rape, torture, acts of organized violence, physical abuse, including witnessing such events, and are therefore likely to suffer psychologically as a result of this exposure. However, this will be dealt with in a separate chapter, as culture can be an important mediator in terms of the manifestation and presentation of post-traumatic reactions.

Therefore, how do post-traumatic stress reactions develop and what maintains the symptoms, such as re-experiencing the event, high levels of anxiety and the avoidance that is often a significant problem for many?

Why do some people develop PTSD and some do not?

It is an intriguing question for many researchers and practitioners as to why some people will go on to develop psychological problems and PTSD following exposure to traumatic events and others do not. This is where an understanding of risk factors is helpful. Often, the stressful or traumatic event itself is rarely enough to produce problems in many of those exposed. A case in point here would be emergency service workers and others exposed to, what for many would be, extreme, harrowing traumatic stressors on a daily or weekly basis, yet often do not go on to develop problems. We will return to some of these issues later.

In general, there are three main categories of risk factors and these are:

◆ pre-trauma factors;

◆ peri-traumatic factors, i.e. specific phenomenon which occur around the time of the event;

◆ post-traumatic factors—these can also be described as complicating factors, as there are a number of issues that can arise following exposure to the traumatic event and serve to exacerbate the individual or family's psychological journey in the wake of the traumatic event.

Whilst a number of risk factors have been identified, the specific risk factors are often not as clearcut as it would seem. In a number of cases, many do not have any pre-trauma risk factors previously identified, yet still go on to develop a range of post-traumatic symptoms and PTSD following exposure to a traumatic event. These are related specifically to the peri-traumatic risk factors and are often concerned with the individual's idiosyncratic meaning of their experience.

Pre-trauma risk factors

Whilst a number of pre-trauma risk factors have been identified, the most significant would be:

◆ Previous stressors—these could also be described as 'life events', such as bereavement, ongoing relationship difficulties, ill-health, work-related stress and financial difficulties.

◆ Previous psychological problems—these could range from previous episodes of anxiety, depression, a family history psychiatric problems, previous history of trauma and childhood abuse.

Peri-traumatic risk factors

These are factors which occur *around the time* of the traumatic event and consist of the following:

◆ The person experiences a sense of loss of control over themselves or events around the time of the trauma.

- Subjective life threat—this refers to the common experience that many people have when exposed to a severe or significant traumatic event, which is that they are going to die.

- The event would involve—exposure to death, serious injury to the individual or a near miss.

- Guilt—there are usually two forms of guilt: one is related to what is often described as 'acts of commission or omission', in other words the individual will perceive, often erroneously, that they did or did not do something, which then led to the event occurring, or to someone coming to some harm; the other form of guilt is known as 'survivor guilt', whereby the individual feels guilt at surviving the experience, whereas a loved one, colleague, friend or others did not.

- Peri-traumatic dissociation—this is a phenomenon that can occur when individuals are exposed to high levels of threat. Dissociation can be described as a range of processes that involve 'the destruction of the usually integrated feelings of consciousness, memory, identity and perception of the environment' (American Psychiatric Association 1994). This is often characterized by individuals describing phenomena, such as 'time having stood still', 'it seemed like it went on forever, but it must have been a few seconds'.

Perhaps the best way of describing the experience of peri-traumatic dissociation is to give two examples. The following is from the explorer David Livingstone, who described his reactions when engaged in shooting a lion.

> When in the act of ramming down the bullets I heard a shout, and looking half round I saw the lion in the act of springing upon me. He caught me on the shoulder and we came to the ground together. Growling horribly he shook me as a dog does a rat. The shock produced a stupor similar to that that seems to be felt by a mouse after the first grip of the cat. It caused a sort of dreaminess in which there was no sense of pain or feeling of terror, although I was quite conscious of all that was happening....

A woman who had been involved in a train crash, where there had been a number of fatalities and injuries, also described a similar phenomenon as follows.

> I was aware of someone on top of me as I couldn't move but I felt no pain and was euphoric and quite elated, even though I had a head wound. I wasn't aware of anybody else on the train only when I looked over my shoulder and saw this pile of bodies....

Another form of peri-traumatic dissociation can be found in Eric Lomax's account of his experiences as a Japanese prisoner of war in Burma:

> At the worst moments I became completely separated from my inner world of pain and sleeplessness. Once I came out into the yard, after what I thought was an all night interrogation and saw the dawn light oiling the

river at the end of the yard, filling our cages with luminous shadow. Suddenly it went dark and I realised I had been watching the sunset.

Here Lomax is describing his disorientation in terms of his altered sense of time following his interrogation at the hands of his captors. Thus, it is very common for individuals to develop a range of post-traumatic reactions and even PTSD where there have been no previous risk factors. The actual event and the meaning of the event, i.e. the individual thinking were going to die and not in control of the situation. They may also have experienced strong feelings of guilt or peri-traumatic dissociation, which were the most significant contributory factors and cause of their difficulties over time.

Post-traumatic risk factors

As indicated previously, these can be described as complicating factors and can influence the outcome of an individual's psychological recovery. These can include a whole range of elements that can often be inter-related.

- Social support—studies have often shown that levels of social support, relatively soon after a traumatic event, can often predict the way symptoms develop over the forthcoming months. Therefore, social support, especially the quality and accessibility of social support, can be a major protective factor following exposure to traumatic events. The type of social support can be informational, practical and emotional, and would vary according to individual needs over time. It is important to match this provision to those needs of individuals, families or communities.

- Substance misuse—the use of alcohol and drugs in the immediate aftermath of a traumatic event in order to deal with the impact can also impact upon, and affect, the recovery process.

- Acute stress reactions or acute stress disorder (ASD)—as indicated in earlier chapters, an acute response following exposure to a traumatic event has been shown to be predictive of problems in the longer term.

There may also be financial considerations, often linked to physical injury, requiring frequent hospital visits, surgery and a loss or change of employment. A perceived lack of justice in the wake of a traumatic event, which can be caused by the way the individual is dealt with by their employer, a social agency or even by a range of historical, social and political events, such as those experienced by many following the Troubles in Northern Ireland, as one example. While the political situation has changed dramatically in Northern Ireland over the past decade, for many there remains feelings of guilt, shame, anger and rage at the events that took place.

Let us also take the example of a major disaster. The scale and the role of the media can often impact upon an individual's recovery, as there will often be frequent reminders through the written and visual media, through documentaries or newspaper and magazine articles. Often people are asked to give interviews about their experiences and these have the potential to harm in perhaps subtle and less obvious ways than first imagined. For example, their stories and experiences may be misrepresented because of factual inaccuracies. They may also be exposed to other aspects of their experience, which may serve to re-traumatize them when they are at their most vulnerable. Accumulative traumatic events can also be seen as another complicating factor, as the individual's exposure to repeated events, which may take their toll over time, finally culminating in an experience that was ultimately too much for them to deal with. People often say things like it was the 'straw that broke the camel's back', meaning that they were managing despite all that had happened and then something else happened. Often it may have been an event they would have normally coped with, but it just added to the weight of everything else, thus affecting their capacity to cope. Often there may be no obvious risk factors present, but the individual develops problems because of various factors that occur after the event, as in the example of Jill's story.

Jill's story

Jill was a passenger in a train crash. She was a 38-year old happily married professional and was 39 weeks pregnant. She had no pre-trauma vulnerabilities.

During the crash, Jill wedged herself on her back between a seat and table fearing that, if the violently shaking train window shattered, she would fall through it and die horribly. On arrival at the hospital, A&E staff could not find the baby's heartbeat, although an experienced midwife later did. She then spent 24 hours strapped to a monitor listening for a change in the baby's heartbeat, which might indicate placental damage. In the event, her baby was born healthy and normally, two weeks later. But she spent those two weeks fearing her baby was dying; she took her concerns to midwives who checked for the unborn baby's health but did not pick up on Jill's growing anxiety. Once her baby was born, she started having nightmares (including 'out of body' experiences) about her baby being dead or them both being trapped in wreckage (which had not happened in the crash).

These nightmares spilled over into her waking life; she saw danger everywhere. She suffered debilitating feelings of sorrow when terrible events happened to other people and gradually she could not cope with the world. She became very withdrawn and, utterly exhausted, was signed-off sick for a few weeks. She returned to work, which in hindsight she knows was far too early and ended up taking a second period of sick leave.

She had a strong belief that, as she was not physically injured, she should just 'get over it' and 'get back on the horse'. So, for about 18 months after the crash, she tried to continue travelling on trains but was effectively re-traumatized on each occasion. She saw an admission that she had been affected by the crash as evidence she was 'not a strong person' and had a 'weak character'.

She now refers to these views as a prejudice (but one she felt is deeply entrenched in a very 'British attitude') that contributed to her withdrawal. Eighteen months after the crash, she began weekly counselling, which initially focused on helping her accept that she had been injured, albeit psychologically, and overcoming her feelings of shame. (We will return to Jill's story in chapter 5)

The assessment

For many trauma sufferers, the assessment process is a difficult and painful process. They will have to discuss events, experiences and memories they have been trying to avoid, often sometimes for many years. However, it is the responsibility of clinicians to treat them with great sensitivity and address their concerns about the process. The therapist needs to acknowledge that the assessment may cause the individual significant discomfort and should reassure them that it is an 'information-gathering' process. The assessment will enable the therapist to find out as much about the trauma and the impact it is having on the individual's life, in order to be able to help the individual try and make sense of, and come to terms with, their experience. Once that information has been gathered (and this may take more than one appointment), appropriate therapy should be discussed. The patient should be given plenty of opportunity to discuss what is on offer in the way of therapy and whether or not they feel it is the right approach for them at that time in their lives.

At this point it must be said that there are different therapeutic approaches to helping trauma sufferers and that therapists with different orientations will approach the assessment process differently. Within the context of this chapter, the assessment approach described will be that of cognitive behaviour therapy (CBT), which is recommended in the National Institute of Clinical Excellence in Health (NICE) Guidelines for The Management PTSD in Adults and Children in Primary and Secondary Care. However, this may not suit everyone, and other approaches will also be discussed. The therapist using this model will also use questionnaires to aid the assessment process and these will be discussed later. The assessment is an extremely important initial contact, as it allows the therapist to develop a rapport with the trauma sufferer, gain a thorough understanding of the person, the problem and their journey since the trauma, and whether or not this approach will work for them. The assessment also allows the CBT therapist to make a *formulation* about the person's problem and give a rationale as to why they feel the approach may work, what the therapy will entail and the anticipated or expected outcomes. For example:

- Why this person?
- Why this problem?
- Why now?

The CBT approach is very collaborative in nature and whilst CBT is often challenging and demanding, the importance of establishing a good rapport and relationship cannot be understated. One of the important things the therapist should try to do is to understand what social support the person has in their life. Do they have people who are able to offer them emotional and practical support when needed? The therapist might use a questionnaire like the one in Figure 3.1 to find out and initiate a conversation about support and how the person uses it. Not everyone makes the best use of the support they have available to them. What the therapist should do is to discuss ways in which the person can make better use of their support.

Assessment of post-traumatic stress

Research has highlighted the need for thorough and comprehensive assessment. Many individuals are often referred to specialist psychological therapy or trauma services with the minimum of information. So the referral letters may contain very little information about the nature and impact of their traumatic experience. They may have previously seen a number of mental health professionals (psychiatrists, community psychiatric nurses or social workers), not to mention counsellors or psychotherapists, and described their experience many times over. This may or may not have been of benefit and, indeed, some of the problems may have resolved and others may have worsened. When interviewed about their problems, they may often not display any degree of distress or emotion. However, this can be misleading as, because they may have recounted their experiences many times, it can seem like telling a story. It may be done with a level of detachment and disassociation, which may belie the distressing and debilitating nature of their traumatic experience. Often this may occur simply because they may have never been asked the appropriate questions in the context of (a) the diagnostic criteria for PTSD. (b) or within the framework of the theoretical models underpinning our understanding of the development of post-traumatic reactions and (c) any considerations of complicating factors or co-morbidity (this refers to the presence of other conditions such as depression). Therefore, a multi-faceted approach to assessment is advocated and needs to include the following areas.

Pre-trauma history

- Establish the individual's previous levels of functioning.
- Determine the person's baseline of functioning.
- Examine the common themes of the individuals life struggles or conflicts.

Immediate pre-trauma psychosocial context

It is extremely important to assess the trauma victim's psychosocial context at the time of the trauma, e.g. what was the individual's age and level of development? What life events was the individual dealing with at the time? What was the level of development of the person's family system?

The event and immediate coping responses

- Was it single or multiple trauma?
- Were the traumas clearly delineated incidents?

or

- Was the trauma a culmination of a number of experiences?
- Was trauma human-induced or an act of nature?
- Did it occur to only one individual, the family or a group?

Active/passive role

- Was the person a helpless victim or perceive their actions as such?
- Was he/she active in any way to alter the situation?
- Were there any options for acting differently?
- How do they perceive the meaning and outcome of their actions?

Meaning of the trauma

This is extremely important because traumatic experiences can have specific idiosyncratic meanings for the individual. This would be dependent on a variety of factors, such as thoughts and imagery, etc., at the time the trauma occurred.

Post-trauma psychosocial context

Areas of consideration should be the presence of ongoing stressors (e.g. the individual is acting as the main carer for an elderly, confused relative; is experiencing relationship problems or going through other significant life events), the responses of the family, the community and social agencies.

- Family responses—often the family or close friends of trauma sufferers may not understand what is happening to the loved one or friend. Because no one wishes to cause those close to them further emotional distress, they may unwittingly encourage avoidance of situations, places or people. On the other hand, they may appear to respond unsympathetically, by becoming irritable with the person because they do not understand what is happening to them and perceive their behaviour as unreasonable.
- Responses from social agencies.

Other areas to consider are:

- Were they treated with respect?
- Were they satisfied with treatment?
- Were there elements of secondary victimization? In other words, did they experience other difficulties in the wake of the event, such as problems being re-housed, receiving criminal injuries compensation or have difficulties with receiving insurance entitlements?

An example here is of a young couple who had put their savings into renovating a small terraced cottage in a former mining village. The cottage was on the main road near a sharp bend. One night whilst watching TV, a car containing four teenagers being driven at speed ploughed into the living room of the house after the driver lost control of the vehicle. A young man in the passenger seat died at the scene. The couple not only witnessed this, but it was some considerable time before they were rescued from the house. Later, after repairs were completed, cracks started to appear in the inner walls and the house was deemed unsafe. The insurance company argued that as their house was an old property, they were ineligible to receive compensation for their loss and this led to a protracted and expensive legal dispute.

Assessment of attribution and meaning

- What are their new views of self and the world?
- Are there new personal outlooks in place?
- What does the trauma mean in terms of the individual's plans for the rest of their life?
- Are they focused on the unfairness of the past or on the possibilities of the future?

Assessing strengths and resources

- When does the person feel better, even when it is only the exception and not the rule?
- What thoughts, feelings and behaviours do they have at those times?
- What coping strategies have been tried that were even partially successful?
- What other difficult situations have they overcome in the past?
- What resources were called upon at that time?
- Who do they see as providing them with support in times of difficulty or crisis?

Evaluate the degree to which:

- the person believes a response exists that will alleviate their suffering;
- the person believes it is within their power to perform the response.

It would also be appropriate to ask about alcohol consumption and a typical drinking week, assessing alcohol intake in units. For alcohol and drugs, change in patterns and amounts following the event need to be considered. Similarly, questions should be asked about prescribed or non-prescribed drugs, and information should be sought regarding current or past medication.

At the end of the assessment

An appropriate course of action needs to be considered, depending on the experience and expertise of the therapist. This would be to:

- ◆ Deal immediately with high levels of anxiety or arousal.

- ◆ Offer advice, guidance and education (see Chapter 5), depending on the length of time between the assessment and the trauma, e.g. if within the first 6–8 weeks, then offer follow-up appointments at regular intervals to assess progress. A reasonable time-frame would be at about one month, three months and then six months.

- ◆ If the person is beginning to have difficulty coping and needs more intensive therapeutic intervention, this should be initiated at this point and an onward referral for specialist trauma focused CBT or other therapy as appropriate should be considered.

4

Intervention strategies: prevention

➜ Key points

- Following trauma and adversity, people are often in a state of shock, disbelief, and are confused and disoriented.

- Over the following days, and weeks, people may often continue to be confused and disoriented, and at this point social support from others is important.

- Timing of help is very important; at some points people need information, at other points, emotional support and at other points practical support.

- In the early stages, information, advice, reassurance and guidance about common reactions, the course of these reactions and signposting for further help are what individuals and families often find most helpful.

- Conventional counselling or therapy within the first 6–8 weeks of exposure to a traumatic event is often not indicated or helpful. Professional advice and help should be sought if common reactions do not subside in intensity, frequency or duration. A variety of strategies can be adopted in order to attempt to mitigate against further adverse reactions or complications from developing.

Many organizations, e.g. the emergency services, use strategies to assist personnel exposed to extremely stressful incidents.

Helping in the aftermath

There has been an ongoing debate over the past two decades as to how best to help people in the aftermath of trauma and adversity. As we have seen in the earlier chapters, not everyone exposed to a traumatic experience will go on to develop severe and long-lasting problems, but others will. We know that one of the most important differences between people who develop problems and those who don't, is social support; so it seems sensible to try to offer support to people.

There is a strong human desire to assist victims of a trauma and attempt to try to undo or ease their pain and suffering. Many academics, psychologists, psychiatrists and psychotherapists would probably agree that prevention of future problems may not always be possible, but there are strategies and supportive interventions, when used appropriately, which may help individuals (and families) at an early stage. In this chapter we will look at what individuals, families and organizations can do to assist those affected.

We will look at what individuals and families may find helpful, especially following a sudden traumatic bereavement following a road-traffic collision, homicide, natural or man-made disaster. We will also look at what organizations, such as the emergency services, offer employees exposed to trauma in the workplace. Finally, some ideas, thoughts and observations on helpful strategies at an early stage will be outlined.

A brief history of early interventions for trauma

The basic framework was drawn from 'crisis-intervention' theories. The period immediately following exposure to a trauma may be considered to constitute a crisis. A crisis can be seen as a state of temporary destabilization and sometimes breakdown in an individual's ability to cope with usual needs and, as mentioned earlier, problem-solving is affected, as may the ability to process and make sense of new information. So a crisis can be caused by an experience of threat, loss or factors that overwhelm or threaten to overwhelm usual coping responses. A significant influencing factor was work developed by Lindemann following support offered to victims of the Coconut Grove nightclub fire in Boston, Massachusetts in 1944, where over 400 people lost their lives. This work was further developed and broadened by Caplan in the early 1960s to be utilized in more broadly defined potentially stressful or traumatic events.

Many organizations, such as the emergency services, banks following armed robbery, and the military, use methods of early intervention for their personnel. The methods were developed over twenty years ago, but are often slightly modified and tailored to meet individual organizational needs. In particular, techniques known as Critical Incident Stress Management (CISM) and Psychological Debriefing (PD) are commonly used.

Psychological debriefing—a brief historical overview

In the 1980s, the idea of helping people in crisis was taken a stage further and developed by Jeffrey Mitchell as a peer-support intervention for emergency service personnel in the United States. The framework became known (and still is) as Critical Incident Stress Management (CISM). It was further developed and refined over the past two decades and been since clearly described as a 'comprehensive, systematic and integrated multi-component crisis intervention package that enables individuals and groups to receive assessment of need, practical support and follow up following exposure to traumatic events in the workplace. In addition, it facilitates the early detection and treatment of post traumatic and other psychological reactions'.

CISM in its current form was originally designed to provide peer support, education and monitoring of individuals and groups of emergency workers, such as fire-fighters and police officers, exposed to potentially traumatic experiences through the course of their work. Therefore emergency service workers may present differently from other trauma survivors, where a single traumatic event is the primary focus of their fears. The armed forces are also more commonly involved in peacekeeping or humanitarian duties and, as a result, they can be exposed to considerable human suffering, with no immediate threat to themselves, and in this respect are increasingly similar to emergency workers. Typical risk scenarios in emergency workers include:

* Repeated experience of a variety of traumatic incidents that entail varying degrees of a sense of personal threat, often combined with the witnessing of harm or death to others, rather than after a single incident.

* An incident where the individual makes some personal identification with a victim or event.

* Repeated intense exposures over a period of time leading to accumulated risk.

* Major terrorist incidents, disasters with multiple loss of life, especially those including children.

CISM programmes within these organizations comprise a number of elements, which include:

* Pre-crisis education—within and for individuals and groups within organizations.

* Assessment—of the nature, potential and actual impact of the incident on individuals and groups involved.

* Defusing—a brief peer-group support meeting within the first 12–24 hours.

* Critical Incident Stress Debriefing (CISD)—a structured group meeting held 72 hours to 14 days post-incident (see below).

* Specialist follow-up for ongoing psychological therapy support, if necessary—usually provided 'in-house' by organizations or out-sourced where necessary.

Controversy arose because attention was focused upon the Critical Incident Stress Debriefing (CISD) component of CISM. CISD is a structured form of crisis intervention and involves a discussion and review of the traumatic event or critical incident, followed by information, advice and guidance on common reactions to trauma, the course of these reactions and signposting as to where further support will be available, should that be necessary. The term Psychological Debriefing (PD) was coined in 1989 by Atle Dyregrov, a Norwegian psychologist who had developed a similar technique. Dyregrov also defined PD as:

> ...a group meeting arranged for the purpose of integrating profound personal experiences both on the cognitive, emotional and group level, and thus preventing the development of adverse reactions.

Since then the terms (especially in Europe) have become interchangeable. The main difference (apart from the names of some of the later phases) is that Dyregrov places more emphasis on the process of the meeting than does Mitchell. The latter has also been developed within a European context and therefore reflects a different tradition for groups and structure than in the US. The other difference is the use of the word 'psychological', which may in some organizational and cultural contexts have negative connotations. This became the focus of attention for research because it was erroneously perceived that this particular aspect of CISM would (a) prevent the development of post-traumatic stress disorder (PTSD) *per se* and (b) was a 'stand-alone' process. For the purposes of this chapter and for the sake of clarity, the term Psychological Debriefing (PD) will be used rather than Critical Incident Stress Debriefing, as it has been widely described as such in the literature and was also used as the working title of the British Psychological Society's Report on Psychological Debriefing.

The most common technique of PD is a structure meeting, facilitated through a series of seven phases of psychological debriefing:

◆ Introduction.

◆ Facts.

◆ Thoughts.

◆ Reactions.

◆ Normalization.

◆ Future planning and coping.

◆ Disengagement.

PD typically takes 1.5–3.0 hours to facilitate and is usually held 72 hours to 14 days post-incident. The aim of PD is to:

◆ Provide education about common reactions to traumatic events and the course of these reactions.

◆ Assist individuals begin the process of coming to terms with the incident / event.

◆ Indicate resources for further help and support, if and where necessary, and facilitate early help seeking, if appropriate.

◆ Facilitate and promote recovery; enhance natural resilience and personal growth.

PD was never intended as a 'stand-alone' intervention or as a substitute for counselling or psychotherapy. It is also often suggested that PD is of little benefit or a 'suitable treatment' for those suffering from PTSD, which is of course true. The reason why PD would be of little benefit is that it was never intended to be used with PTSD sufferers. It was intended as an educative crisis intervention strategy, to be used for emergency services personnel, e.g. fire-fighters, paramedics, police officers and similar occupational groups, within the first 2–4 weeks following their exposure to an incident that would have been assessed to have the potential to impact upon their mental health and well-being. As we have seen earlier, *PTSD can only be diagnosed one month after exposure to the traumatic event.*

You will see that these methods of debriefing are about providing people with information, guidance and advice as to what to expect. Certainly, for some people, at certain points, this is extremely valuable to do. But, PD is not a form of therapy for the treatment of post-traumatic stress. Sometimes, the media has created confusion by labelling it as 'counselling'.

Current use of CISM and PD within organizations

Current evidence at the time of writing, suggests that many organizations, especially the emergency services and some sections of the military in the UK and abroad, continue to utilize CISM and PD as part of their post-incident support measures for personnel. Around the late-1980s, London's Metropolitan Police and many other police forces in the UK utilized PD, but adapted the technique from Mitchell and Dyregrov, which became known as the three-stage model, comprising of:

- Facts (equating to the Introduction and Facts phase of PD).
- Feelings (equating to Thoughts and Reactions phase of PD).
- Future (equating to Normalization, Future Planning/Coping and Disengagement phases of PD).

Whilst this adaptation of the technique was in use for a number of years, the current focus is to re-train many peer-support teams in CISM/PD using Dyregrov's approach. In view of the past controversy and the NICE guidelines, there has also been a trend for some organizations to develop new CISM models. As a result, CISM still continues to be used by a number of organizations but is referred to in a variety of different ways. Below are a number of new terms that describe the CISM process. For example:

- Critical Incident Processing(CIPR)—which contains all the CISM elements recommended and described above.
- Trauma Risk Management (TRiM)—developed by two mental health professionals for the British Royal Marines, it is described as a post-traumatic management strategy, based upon peer-group assessment for hierarchical organizations.

It also contains all the CISM components and utilizes the three-stage technique of PD.

◆ Emotional Decompression—a relatively recent addition, it is also is a hybrid of the three-stage technique and seven-stage PD technique.

Therefore, on closer inspection, models that purport to be offering different solutions to post-trauma support in the workplace are all practicing CISM and PD under new acronyms. It also means that many organizations are offering similar post-incident support systems but modifying the process to suit their organizational context and needs, such as TRiM, which is well-suited to a military context.

The research and current recommendations

There are only two studies that have suggested that CISM and PD may not be helpful and have promoted the idea that it has the potential to cause harm. These studies, however, were conducted with hospitalized individuals who had experienced a road-traffic collision or a burn trauma. They were not conducted with groups that the interventions were originally intended for, and have been the source of much debate and controversy in the field, as mentioned above. It has also been recognized that the studies have methodological flaws; further research is needed. It was also noted in the NICE guidelines, that none of the studies that showed negative effects contained any descriptions of the training given to those carrying out the interventions, as these involve a different set of skills. There are nevertheless a number of studies that have also shown CISM/PD to be helpful, well-accepted by those receiving the intervention and that CISM/PD does not cause harm. Thus, when it is used in high-risk occupational settings, such as the emergency services, the aims are usually as follows:

◆ A practical means of providing social and organizational support.

◆ Helps contextualize the traumatic experience

◆ Facilitates emotional processing (the 're-packing of the bag').

◆ Helps challenge perception of guilt and self-blame, where present.

◆ Facilitates and encourages the use of appropriate coping strategies.

◆ Facilitates early help seeking—thus hopefully preventing possible psychological complications in the longer term.

◆ Helps to diminish the impact of the traumatic event.

The reasons for providing social support are based on overwhelming evidence from 30 years of research that it is a major protective factor following major life events or trauma. There are different types of social support:

◆ Informational, practical and emotional.

◆ The type of social support required depends on the context and individual needs.

- These will vary over time.
- It is important to match support provision to needs.

Wherever it is offered, it is not the aim or intention to prevent or reduce symptoms of PTSD, but as a means of providing social support. There are numerous other examples where early interventions are offered to provide practical, emotional and social support following exposure to traumatic events. In these cases what is offered will *not be* psychological debriefing, but often the general principles of support offered is the same. The most notable example was following the Tsunami of 2005. Since then the Foreign and Commonwealth Office has worked closely with the British Red Cross to provide psychosocial support to UK nationals affected by incidents abroad. The British Red Cross Psychosocial Support Team (PST) consists of professionals drawn from a variety of settings, both within the British Red Cross and externally from organizations such as social services and the NHS with a health, mental health and social care background.

In summary, therefore, the fundamental guidelines for early support that should be followed when working with individuals and groups after exposure to traumatic events, and those that are at the core of CISM and PD offered by numerous organizations, are:

- Early support should be based on good assessment.
- Provide pragmatic psychological support in an empathic manner, provide information about common reactions, course of these reactions, advice on coping strategies and 'signpost' for further help.
- Individuals who show a continued increase in the frequency, intensity and duration of any common or adverse reactions should be offered/may benefit from formal intervention.
- An approach that takes account of an individual's natural resilience.
- Attendance at support meetings should be voluntary.

The process of recovery

Just as there are many normal ways of reacting to traumatic experiences, so too there are many ways of dealing with the impact of these events. One way of understanding this, is to consider the following analogy.

When someone is exposed to, or experiences, a traumatic event, they often experience a range of thoughts and emotions that they are unable to deal with, or make sense of, at the time of the trauma, for various reasons. For example, they may be frightened, shocked or numb, in pain, worried about loved ones, being cut out of a car, being interviewed by the police. As a result, these thoughts or emotions are often hurriedly 'packed' in an imaginary bag and taken away with them from the scene of the trauma. However, this 'emotional luggage', because it has been hurriedly and not well packed, may frequently burst open from time to time or when it is 'knocked against' something. This is often experienced as distressing thoughts, images, nightmares and other emotions, which they have tried to push out of their mind because they find them so upsetting. Common examples would be when they are exposed to situations or events that resemble aspects of the trauma or the trauma itself.

What many people do over time is unpack and repack their bag, thereby helping themselves to come to terms with, and make sense of, their traumatic experience. Inevitably there are things they have to keep, e.g. the traumatic experience. Eventually they will be able to dispense with many items, e.g. guilt, anger, and re-arrange others; this might involve them having different perceptions of their experience. The aim is to eventually be able to carry the bag without it bursting open unexpectedly, and that they can open it and view the contents at any time without undue distress. In addition, because this act of 'bursting open' is happening much less frequently, the bag becomes hardly noticeable. However, whilst the unpacking and repacking is a painful process, this becomes easier over time. Ways of facilitating this process are discussed below.

'Natural' forms of self protection

Some of the reactions to trauma are in themselves ways of protecting a person and of coping with distressing experiences. These include:

- ◆ Numbness. You may find that initially your feelings seem blocked off and that the event seems very distant or dream-like. This can be a way of allowing the distress of the incident to be felt only slowly and gradually. Others around you may (wrongly) think you are 'unfeeling' or 'being strong'.
- ◆ Going over the event. Letting the experience enter your mind and thinking about it can allow you to try to make sense of what has happened.

Things you can do to promote recovery—a few self-help strategies to consider

Susan was driving her car on a major motorway during the early evening, returning from work. She was involved in a collision after a car overtook at speed, colliding with a heavy goods vehicle which was behind her. The resulting collision involved her car being spun across the carriageway facing into the path of oncoming cars. She was not injured but badly shaken and had to be released by the Fire Service from the car, which took almost 30 minutes. She was taken to hospital but released home in a few hours in the care of her husband. She took three days off work, as suggested by her manager, but returned using a courtesy car. Initially she was naturally apprehensive when driving but this apprehension began to increase gradually in a space of a few days. She soon found that she was taking opportunities to avoid driving on dual carriageways and motorways, and then began avoiding relatively short journeys. She soon started to become apprehensive and anxious even at the thought of driving or being a passenger. Within four weeks of the accident she had almost stopped altogether and this inevitably affected her work and social life. She would avoid talking about it and started to gradually cut herself off from friends and extended family.

In Susan's case, her understandable avoidance and anxiety in the early stages were adaptive. However, her gradual mental and behavioural avoidance only served to maintain and worsen her problem. If you, a loved one or friend, has recently been through a traumatic event, e.g. a road-traffic collision (RTC), experienced an assault, witnessed an accident, say within the past few weeks and have experienced some or many of what have been described earlier as common reactions to such events, it may be worth considering or suggesting some of the following to promote recovery.

Accessing and accepting support from others

It is very comforting to receive physical and emotional support from other people. It is important not to reject support by trying to appear strong, or trying to cope completely on your own. Talking to others who have had similar experiences, or who understand what you have been through, is particularly important. It can allow you to release pent-up feelings and enable barriers to come down and closer relationships to develop. Some friends may be reluctant to offer their support, even though they would like to help—do not be afraid to ask and say what you want. There is overwhelming evidence that has shown that social support is a major protective factor following exposure to traumatic events or significant life crises. This will also enhance the natural resilience of individuals, families and communities.

Monitor your reactions over time. The most important consideration is to watch out for any avoidance behaviour, as described earlier. It is often very common for people who have been through a traumatic experience to want to avoid thoughts, places, activities or people who may remind them in some way of their experience. Given the wide range of traumatic experiences that a person may encounter, this can be an extensive list. However, if this continues, it almost always leads to further problems in the longer term. Therefore, it is helpful to encourage the person to gradually begin to face fearful situations. The simplest way to do this is to try small steps gradually increasing the frequency and duration of the exposure to the feared situation. It is often said that the best way to deal with situations, as in Susan's case above, is 'to get back on the horse'. The important factor here is how one 'gets back on the horse', because doing too much too soon can be detrimental and be aversive. Therefore, some simple stages for somebody who has been in an RTC would be to:

- Just sit in the car.
- Sit in the car with the engine running.
- Drive very short distances in familiar settings, e.g. down the street and back.
- Increase driving time and distances in familiar settings.
- Drive on familiar roads in quiet times.
- Drive on familiar roads at busy times.

As can be seen, this could be extended as necessary; however, there are some very simple but important rules that should be followed for exposure to feared situations to be effective and these are: activities should be often enough, frequent enough and above all there should be consistency.

Taking time out for yourself

In order to deal with their feelings, some people find it necessary at times to be alone, or just be with close friends or family. Sometimes this can be difficult when we lead busy lives and we have to negotiate carefully with our friends and family to make space for ourselves.

Confronting what has happened

Confronting the reality of the situation, e.g. by talking to a close friend, colleague or confidante, will help individuals to come to terms with the event. This can be the hardest thing, to accept the reality of our losses, and to face up to the way in which our life has changed. But although this is important, it's also important to recognize that everyone has their own ways and speed of doing this, and we should not try to rush people.

Staying active

Helping others, keeping busy and engaging in previously enjoyed activities can give some temporary relief. Physical activity is really beneficial to our psychological well-being. Research has shown that 30 minutes of activity a day, e.g., walking, gardening, etc., can have a positive effect on mood. So we would recommend strongly that people manage to maintain their activity levels. Often we won't feel like it following trauma, and so it requires that little bit extra effort. It can be simple things, like taking the stairs when you would rather take the lift, walking instead of taking the car. Even if you take exercise in periods of a few minutes, say 10–20 minutes at a time, that is still useful.

Returning to usual and familiar routines

It is usually advisable to return to usual routines as soon as possible after the event in order to avoid incubation and magnification of fear while away from the situation. While it is important to try to return to our routines because of those benefits, people will have different speeds at which they can do this.

New interests

There is also a window of opportunity following trauma to make new changes in life. For example, taking up new activities, interests and socializing, can be helpful to people in the recovery process.

All of the above can prove very helpful and make your experience easier to bear. However, over-use of some coping mechanisms can be counter-productive and even detrimental if they divert you from getting the help and support you need. Over-activity or excessive use of distraction can, for example, be unhelpful if it prevents you confronting the reality of the event. Your recovery may be delayed if you suppress your feelings too much or for too long (numbness), or if you become preoccupied with repeated thoughts of the event. Gradually confronting the reality of what has happened, accepting support from others and talking through your feelings are particularly important ways of gaining emotional release and coming to terms with your experiences.

Who should I talk to?

Generally speaking it is 'good to talk' about our reactions and feelings about what has happened. In the main it is probably best to talk to people who you know, trust and feel comfortable with—usually this will be with members of your family or with close friends. Sometimes, however, this may not be possible—you may be away from your family and friends, your family or friends may themselves have been involved, or you may find it difficult to talk about your feelings within your family (because you do not wish to upset them, or because relationships are strained). If this is the case, you might find it helpful to talk to colleagues at work, to your GP, a member of the clergy or seek professional mental health advice and support. Remember though that you do not 'have' to talk to a counsellor or therapist if you don't want to, and that, where possible, it is usually enough to draw upon usual forms of support, your family or significant others.

There are different types of counsellor and psychotherapist available. Cognitive-behavioural counsellors and psychotherapists are very structured and focus on identifying the ways in which your thinking affects your behaviours and emotions, and how by changing your thinking habits you can change how you feel. In trauma, they are also interested in how your behaviour influences how you feel. For example, traumatized people are often very avoidant of fearful situations and so the therapist will encourage people to confront their experiences, either in imagination, or in real life. Other types of therapists may help us understand how childhood shaped us as people, and how by helping us make sense of our pasts we can take more control of our future. Often we become aware of things we weren't previously aware of before. Different therapists will offer different things, but never be scared to ask them about what they are doing. A good therapist will be pleased to explain why they are doing what they are doing.

When to seek professional help

It is important that you allow yourself to talk to your family or friends about your experiences and feelings at the earliest opportunity. If, however, some of the normal reactions described above are particularly intense and distressing, or if they persist or have persisted for a long time (for more than about 6 to 8 weeks), it is advisable to seek professional help, sooner rather than later. Some of the pointers that suggest you should consider asking for help include:

◆ If you feel that you are overwhelmed by, and cannot handle, intense feelings and bodily sensations.

◆ If you have no one to share your emotions with and you feel the need to do so.

◆ You continue to feel numb and empty, or have persistent feelings of tension, confusion, exhaustion or other unpleasant bodily sensations.

◆ You have to keep overactive in order not to focus on your feelings.

◆ You want to avoid thoughts, places, activities or people who may remind you in some way, however subtle, of your experience.

◆ You continue to have frequent distressing thoughts or recollections of the traumatic experience.

◆ You continue to have nightmares or poor sleep.

◆ Your relationships seem to be suffering badly, or sexual problems develop.

◆ You are drinking to excess.

◆ Your work performance suffers, you make mistakes or you have accidents associated with poor concentration.

It may be helpful to try the the trauma screening questionnaire (TSQ), which is a self-report scale of individual responses to a traumatic event (Fig. 4.1). It consists of ten questions measuring re-experiencing of the event and symptoms of arousal. It is designed for use a month or more following exposure to a traumatic event, to identify individuals who may be suffering from symptoms of post-traumatic stress. It only take a few minutes to complete and the scoring is simple and straightforward. Answering yes, to six or more items could mean that the person may be at risk of suffering from PTSD and would benefit from further detailed assessment. The time-frame is a month or more following exposure to a traumatic event—it is not designed to be used before that time. It assesses current symptoms and does not diagnose PTSD. It is based on research conducted with train crash survivors.

Other important points to remember

◆ If you have experienced a personal loss as a result of the incident, then this recovery may take considerably longer, e.g. months, sometimes years.

◆ In addition, changes in outlook and attitude towards others and the world are common; these may be lasting and will fluctuate over time, but in most cases they are for the better and the effects are positive. However, if they are becoming problematic, confusing or distressing they can be addressed with professional help.

◆ Anniversaries will be coming up, as will be birthdays and other memorable occasions. Whilst these will be distressing, try and commemorate them in your own way. Inevitably there may be family tensions and disagreements (this is very normal!), aim for compromise and agree to differ. If needs be, hold separate small personal ceremonies.

Please consider the following reactions, which sometimes occur after a traumatic event. This questionnaire is concerned with your personal reactions to the traumatic event that happened to you. **Please indicate (by circling either Yes or No) whether or not you have experienced any of the following at least twice in the past week.**

Upsetting thoughts or memories about the event that have come into your mind against your will	Yes	No
Upsetting dreams about the event	Yes	No
Acting or feeling as though the event were happening again	Yes	No
Feeling upset by reminders of the event	Yes	No
Bodily reactions (such as fast heartbeat, stomach churning, sweatiness, dizziness) when reminded of the event	Yes	No
Difficulty falling or staying asleep	Yes	No
Irritability or outbursts of anger	Yes	No
Difficulty concentrating	Yes	No
Heightened awareness of potential dangers to yourself and others	Yes	No
Being jumpy or being startled at something unexpected	Yes	No

Figure 4.1 The Trauma Screening Questionnaire (TSQ). Brewin C.R. et al (2002). Reproduced with permission from the *British Journal of Psychiatry*, **181**, 158–162.

Some do's and don'ts to remember
DO

- Express your emotions, take the opportunity to review the experience within yourself and with others, let your family share in your experiences.
- Express your needs clearly and honestly to your family, friends and managers and colleagues at work.
- Take time out to sleep, rest, think and be with your close family and friends.
- Try to keep your life as normal as possible after the initial period of often intense acute distress.

DON'T

◆ Bottle up feelings, avoid talking about what has happened, or let your embarrassment stop you giving others the chance to talk.

◆ Expect the memories to go away quickly—they may stay with you for some time.

◆ Forget that if others are involved they may be experiencing similar feelings to you.

Whilst people often say that after a traumatic event 'Things will never be the same again...', to some extent this may be true but do remember that you are basically the same person that you were before the incident and that if you feel unable to cope with your feelings and reactions, support and advice is available.

Where to seek professional help

If you wish to find out more about the availability of confidential counselling you should in the first instance approach your own GP, who will be able to advise you on options and put you in touch with someone who can help. This may be:

◆ A counsellor in the GP surgery.

◆ A mental health professional from the local community mental health team (psychiatrist community mental health nurse, social worker, psychologist, specialist therapist or occupational therapist).

◆ Some areas have specialist trauma and bereavement services and these can be accessed by your GP.

◆ If there are no specialist services locally, your local Primary Care Trust (PCT) can fund you to attend specialist services for assessment and treatment in another part of the country.

Other options are to seek support from organizations such as Cruse and Victim Support (there is a list at the end of the book in other countries this will differ and in some cases it may be provided by organisations such as the Red Cross). You may wish to seek help privately from a therapist or counsellor. Don't hesitate to ask them about their experience, qualifications and, most importantly, their experience of working with psychological trauma or traumatic bereavement. This is especially important if you are seeing them in the early stages after experiencing an event; say within the first 4–6 weeks. Also if you are seen within that time-frame, ensure you are offered a follow-up appointment. In addition, if you decide to pursue this as an avenue of help, it is important to find someone with whom you feel comfortable and safe.

Conclusion

Deciding whether an individual is experiencing problems or a range of reactions that will spontaneously resolve after a traumatic event can be difficult. Understanding and being aware of the psychological trajectory of the response within the first 6–8 weeks can be helpful in determining the probable course of their reactions. If the initial distress is steadily diminishing in frequency, intensity and duration, then there is every chance that recovery and a return to what for them would be stability and equilibrium. However, if the reactions persist or are increasingly problematic, advice, guidance and support should be sought. A mental health assessment may be appropriate to assess and determine individual needs, with attention being paid to a risk assessment and other factors, such as previous vulnerabilities and social support. Information from relatives can also be an important part of this process. Interventions that include education, advice and guidance, based on and related to their unique experience, can be helpful. Follow-up is important to assess progress over the following months.

5

Treatment for post-traumatic stress

> ## ⟳ Key points
>
> ◆ Severe PTSD can be effectively treated with trauma-focused psychological interventions such as cognitive behavioural therapy (CBT).
>
> ◆ Medication should not usually be used as first line of treatment for PTSD sufferers, but may be helpful if (a) the person does not respond to psychological approaches and (b) lives under serious current threat of further trauma. Medications, especially anti-depressants, are often helpful as an adjunct to psychological treatment.
>
> ◆ Medication should *not* be used with children and adolescents to treat PTSD.
>
> ◆ Eye movement desensitization and reprocessing (EMDR) can be an effective treatment technique for treatment of PTSD.
>
> ◆ Other psychological treatment approaches may also be helpful to people who have experienced trauma, depending on individual needs.
>
> ◆ Existential and humanistic therapies can also help people to come to terms with changes in their lives.
>
> ◆ Litigation can often affect the course of psychological treatment.

Introduction

As we have seen, common post-traumatic stress reactions can in some cases develop into the chronic and disabling condition we have described in detail earlier as post-traumatic stress disorder (PTSD). Furthermore, there is not only a significant impact on the individual, but also on their partners, families and relationships in general. Their ability to work, socialize and lead active, productive lives and contribute to society, as they previously did, may be seriously affected, often for many years. In addition, secondary mental health problems, such as depression, anxiety, panic attacks, phobias and alcohol and drug abuse, can also complicate the problem. Financial hardship, social isolation and the breakdown or loss of support networks are also common. Physical injury (this will be explored in more detail in Chapter 7) and personal losses can serve to further complicate matters. Usually many sufferers present to their GP months and sometimes years after the trauma. However, even when they do seek help earlier, PTSD may go unrecognized. A research survey conducted after the 7/7 London bombings suggested that PTSD may be under-recognized in primary care settings. This result was in keeping with a similar earlier study with 7/7 survivors and studies conducted in other countries, which have shown that PTSD is often under-recognized in public mental health services. There may be a variety of reasons why this low recognition occurs, which may include the following:

- Time constraints and lack of information in GP surgeries.

- PTSD sufferers may be reluctant to inform their GP, as they often find talking about their experience extremely distressing.

- People suffering the effects of a traumatic experience may not be aware of the condition of PTSD.

- Sufferers often do not understand what is happening (as in Laura's story previously), but have developed unhelpful coping strategies, such as avoidance of reminders of the event, and this may include not seeking help for fear of having to discuss their experiences.

- Press and media coverage often represents the impact of traumatic experiences on individuals in a simplistic way, misrepresenting or confusing facts about the condition or the interventions used, often suggesting that help-seeking is a sign of weakness, as characterized by the article headline in one major Sunday newspaper, which read, 'A stiff upper lip beats stress counselling'.

- Many feel they have to overcome their problems on their own.

- Many feel ashamed over the event and their responses.

- Children and adolescents may hide symptoms from parents.

- Many are not aware that PTSD is a treatable condition.

Of course, the longer the condition continues, the more chronic and intense the symptoms become. The mental and behavioural avoidance becomes more entrenched, sleep becomes more disturbed, often with disturbing dreams, irritability, concentration and physical symptoms become more marked. Relationship difficulties deepen and other emotional states, such as anger, guilt, sadness and emotional numbing, are ever present. Sometimes the more chronic and disabling the symptoms, the more difficult the road to recovery can be. However, it must be emphasized that this should not put anyone off from seeking help, as the length of time between the trauma and receiving help can make a difference to treatment outcome, because (a) everyone is different, (b) there are effective treatment techniques and strategies that work and (c) there is nothing to be lost by exploring what help might be right for you.

What sort of professional help is the most effective?

There are many forms of 'talking therapies' and you should ask your therapist or counsellor to describe and explain the type of therapy they offer, what it involves, how long it will last and what the research evidence is for the type of technique or therapy they use. Many types of therapy can be helpful and talking to a therapist can be very helpful.

There is considerably less orthodoxy in the fields of counselling, psychotherapy, psychology and psychiatry than in general medicine where, for example, there is generally an agreement on the methods of treatment of many medical conditions, with minor differences in the application of treatment and management of the condition. However, when it comes to mental health, there is a greater variability on therapeutic methods and who offers which therapy. Counsellors, psychotherapists, psychologists and psychiatrists are all involved in offering help, but each profession has its own language and way of thinking, and it can therefore be confusing. As a consequence, psychological/psychotherapeutic interventions can and do vary considerably, often depending on the type of approach the counsellor or therapist uses.

This then begs the question of which psychotherapeutic option is likely to be the most effective for PTSD. Whilst the contribution of psychoanalytic thinking to our understanding of the development PTSD should be acknowledged, there are no outcome studies to indicate the effectiveness of psychoanalytic or psychodynamic therapy for PTSD. In addition, despite the rapid growth of counsellors, especially within primary care, there is little evidence that generic counselling, provided by itself, is particularly effective in the treatment of PTSD.

Often when someone is suffering from PTSD, and the situation is beginning to affect the individual's social and occupational functioning, more active, practical forms of intervention are helpful. Research suggests that a type of psychological therapy, known as cognitive behavioural therapy (CBT) can be very effective. It is especially effective for the treatment of psychological trauma and for those individuals suffering from PTSD; this will be described in more detail later in the chapter.

Current treatment recommendations

The National Institute for Clinical Excellence in Health (NICE) in the UK is an independent organization responsible for providing national guidance and promoting good health and the treatment of specific clinical conditions. In addition, it produces clinical practice guidelines, derived from the best available research evidence, using pre-determined and systematic methods to identify and evaluate all the evidence in relation to the specific condition in question. Where it is considered that this evidence is lacking, the guidelines aim to incorporate statements and recommendations based upon the consensus statements developed by the guidelines' group. The NICE guidelines for *Post-traumatic Stress Disorder (PTSD): The Management of PTSD in Adults and Children in Primary and Secondary Care* were published in 2005 and were developed to advise on the treatment and management of PTSD. Guideline recommendations were developed by a multi-disciplinary team of healthcare professionals, guideline methodologists and PTSD sufferers, after consideration of the best available evidence. The intention is that these NICE guidelines (along with others) would be useful to clinicians and service commissioners in providing a high quality of care to PTSD sufferers, including emphasis on the importance of the experience of carers.

The NICE guidelines for PTSD provide a comprehensive review on the current best practice in the assessment and management of PTSD in primary and secondary care. The intention is that once the national guidelines have been published and disseminated, local healthcare providers will be expected to produce plans and identify resources with its implementation along with appropriate timetables. The intention is that multi-disciplinary health groups, involving commissioners, specialist mental health professionals, patients and carers would undertake the translation of the implementation to local protocols. Ultimately, the nature and time-frame of any local plans reflect upon local needs and the nature of existing provisions

Trauma-focused psychological therapy

The NICE guidelines recommend that PTSD sufferers should be offered a course of trauma-focused psychological therapy, typically this would mean trauma-focused cognitive behaviour therapy (CBT), which may often include eye movement desensitization and reprocessing (EMDR) (described below) and other techniques. CBT is conducted over a relatively short space of time, usually 8–12 individual treatment sessions, over a period of months. It is an active and directive form of therapy, aimed at teaching individuals how to confront and eventually overcome their fears, avoidances and anxious thoughts. All cognitive behavioural methods are:

- Structured and directive in nature.
- Problem and technique orientated.
- Directed toward helping the individual achieve their goals.
- Collaborative.
- Focused on the 'here and now'.
- Based upon use of explicit, agreed treatment strategies.

Techniques also include helping the sufferer challenge and change problematic thoughts and meanings about the trauma, which may include feelings of guilt or loss of trust in others. CBT also includes exposure therapy. Exposure therapy helps the individual confront feared reminders and memories of the trauma in a graded way (i.e. taking a step at a time). Like any form of therapy, it can be challenging, because the individual will have to confront situations they have been avoiding, often for a considerable time. It is a very human response to want to avoid pain at any cost, whether physical or emotional. Exposure to reminders and memories can be painful, but with help, encouragement and support many PTSD sufferers can come to terms with traumatic experiences.

Pierre Janet's therapeutic approach to traumatized patients was the first attempt to create a systematic, phase-orientated treatment of post-traumatic stress. Janet viewed the trauma response as a disorder of memory that interfered with effective action. He also believed, and taught, that effective treatment consisted of the importance of forming a stable therapeutic relationship, which would facilitate the retrieving and transforming of traumatic memories into meaningful experiences and taking effective action to overcome learned helplessness. Janet's belief that a good, safe therapeutic relationship—what he described as a 'rapport' between patient and therapist—was indispensible for resolution of the trauma. Whilst not everyone may achieve resolution of all their difficulties, his thinking about therapeutic relationships remains relevant today.

Cognitive behavioural therapy (CBT)

Exposure to reminders and memories of the trauma remain common to most approaches, but in CBT exposure is conducted in a systematic way, based upon research that these approaches can be effective. Different aspects of CBT approaches to trauma are described below.

Assessment

This is an extremely important process before therapy begins and some of the areas that are addressed in assessment were covered in Chapter 3. However, in addition to the assessment interview, patients are also asked to fill in self-report questionnaires, such as the TSQ on page 46, which also provide very helpful information and are used to form a baseline, monitor progress, either session by session or at the end of therapy and at follow-up. These are relatively straightforward to fill out and if there is any difficulty ask a relative, friend or the therapist to help. They provide a snap-shot of specific aspects of the individual's traumatic experience, such as the frequency of intrusive thoughts, avoidance, mood, sleep, concentration and so on. The most common are described below, but there are others that may be used by the therapist to highlight or focus on areas they feel may be of benefit in therapy; one such example is the Changes in Outlook Questionnaire (CiOQ). The CiOQ is shown in Chapter 8. Another tool that may help clients identify change is the Psychological Well-being Post-Trauma Changes Questionnaire (PWB-PTCQ) which we have developed to assess changes in self-acceptance, autonomy, mastery, purpose in life, relationships and personal growth (see Appendix 2). This is a short easy to use tool which therapist's may find useful alongside the more traditional measures of post traumatic stress, which we will now turn to.

Interviews

The clinician-administered PTSD scale DSM IV (CAPS) (Blake *et al.* 1995)

This is a well-validated instrument and is seen as a 'gold standard' diagnostic tool, which was developed to measure cardinal and hypothesized signs and symptoms of PTSD. It is not a self-report measure and is carried out as an interview by the therapist with the patient. The interview can be a lengthy process, taking over an hour to complete. It provides a method to evaluate the frequency and intensity of individual symptoms, as well as the impact of symptoms in social and occupational functioning, the overall intensity of the symptoms and the validity of the ratings obtained. It also provides an opportunity for the clinician to rate the veracity and accuracy of symptom descriptions, their severity and intensity, thus allowing the overall validity of responses to be assessed. Factors considered are compliance with the interview, mental state, e.g. problems with concentration, comprehension of items, disassociation, and any evidence of efforts to exaggerate or minimize symptoms). Every symptom is rated for frequency (from 0—never to 4—daily or almost every day) and intensity (from 0—none to 4—extreme, incapacitating distress). Where a symptom is positively endorsed, the patient is asked to give a detailed description or example. The time-frame used in the CAPS is a month period prior to interview. The CAPS may often be used if someone is attending for a medico-legal interview, i.e. they are being assessed for a litigation claim following a road-traffic collision or industrial injury. It is not used by all therapists, but is often used in specialist treatment centres.

Self-report questionnaires

We have already seen one tool for assessing post-traumatic stress, the TSQ. Some common self-report questionnaires are listed below. Unlike the CAPS, these questionnaires do not diagnose someone as having PTSD and are not intended or should be used for this purpose. This is not meant as an exhaustive list, but merely as an indication of those in most frequent use.

Impact of event scale (IES) (Horowitz 1979)

This questionnaire is widely used in research and clinical practice following exposure to traumatic events and is a measure of subjective distress in relation to the experience. It has 15 items and two subscales; intrusion/re-experiencing and avoidance. The usual 'cut-off' point is 35. This means that if a person scores 35 or more, they can be seen as having a significant reaction in the moderate-to-severe range. There is also the revised impact of event scale (IES-R), which has 22 items that include the hyper-arousal criteria of PTSD, such as feeling constantly on guard, irritability and anger. Both scales are in common use.

The post-traumatic diagnostic scale (PDS) (Foa 1996)

This questionnaire enquires about PTSD symptoms and is designed to aid in diagnosis based on DSM IV criteria and gives a measure of PTSD symptom severity. The PDS offers respondents a checklist of 12 traumatic events. First, they have to endorse all those events that they have experienced and to define which event has caused them the most distress. Second, respondents then rate each of 17 items corresponding to the 17 DSM-IV symptoms of PTSD. Each of the 17 items is rated on a four-point scale. Finally, respondents are asked questions regarding the duration of symptoms and inquiries regarding impairment in a variety of areas. Like other questionnaires, it is intended to be used in conjunction with a clinical interview and through assessment.

Post-traumatic cognitions inventory (PTCI) (Foa et al. 2007)

This questionnaire attempts to assess particular themes related to the individual's negative beliefs about the self, world and self-blame. In the clinical setting an individual's thoughts and beliefs can be focused on in treatment, and progress and outcome tracked over time.

Beck depression inventory (BDI) (Beck et al. 1961)

This is a well-known and well-validated clinical and research tool. It is a 21-item, self-rating questionnaire, allowing for rapid assessment of depressive symptoms. Sometimes it is administered on a weekly basis.

General health questionnaire-28 (GHQ-28) (Goldberg 1981)

This is a self-rating questionnaire for screening for psychiatric problems in the general population. The threshold/cut-off point for identifying 'psychiatric caseness', i.e. the likelihood that the individual could be classified as having minor mental health problems, is 5. However, if used with someone who has had a physical injury or with more complex problems, it would be more appropriate to raise the threshold/cut-off point to 13 or above.

Cognitive therapy

Cognitive therapy operates on a multi-layered understanding of the relationship between cognitions (thoughts), behaviours, emotion and how these are affected and influenced by an individual's experience; hence it is described as cognitive behavioural therapy, as thoughts, attitudes and beliefs i.e. attitudinal change, can only be brought about through behavioural experience. The model is problem-orientated, focuses on the 'here and now', is active, directive and, most importantly, collaborative. The focus here is on the identification of the shattered beliefs and assumptions, and the rebuilding of these through what is described as 'cognitive restructuring'; in other words, trying to help individuals think differently about the experience and develop new meanings. The CION (see Appendix 1) may be useful in identifying some of these problematic beliefs and how strongly they are held. Trauma-focused cognitive therapy attempts to change problematic meanings of the traumatic experience such as 'What happened shows that I am bad/inferior/ useless person', 'I cannot trust anyone anymore', and changing problematic coping responses, such as thought-suppression, ruminating on negative outcomes or selectively attending to threat.

Graded exposure

Graded exposure, also known as exposure *in vivo* (or real life), involves exposure in real life to feared/avoided situations, either directly related to the traumatic event or which resembled it in some way. This could be either graded or prolonged, and either therapist-aided or unaccompanied. Partners or significant other family members are often encouraged to act as a co-therapist, if possible. Patients are given specific instructions and guidelines for exposure therapy, emphasis being placed on consistency within the treatment programme. A rationale for exposure is often given as below:

> Usually, some anxiety occurs when you start this type of programme. This is actually an important part of treatment, because often people think that the anxiety will continue and become intolerable. One of the valuable things you learn through treatment is that the anxiety does not increase to intolerable levels and it often subsides more rapidly than you might expect. Sometimes, anxiety starts to reduce within 20 minutes; more usually, half an hour to an hour. Another important thing that you will notice is that, after you have done exposure two or three times, the amount of discomfort you get at first becomes less and less. This is the best indication of how the treatment is working; as time goes on, you will find you will be able to do the exposure in this way and get no discomfort at all.

One way of describing the way exposure works, is to consider it a form of 'emotional physiotherapy'. For example, if a person has an accident and injures or breaks a limb, they are often prescribed a course of physiotherapy, which they have to attend regularly and is often painful, sometimes causing some discomfort for some hours afterwards, perhaps even a few days. When done in frequent, regular and repeated sessions, there is a cumulative effect and the distress and discomfort gradually decrease in time. In addition, exercises are also recommended and suggested. In this way, the individual gradually learns to use their limb again. Experience of a case on the burns unit is a good illustration of this idea of emotional physiotherapy.

Chen's story

Chen was a man of Chinese origin, who was receiving treatment on the burns unit after being badly injured in an explosion in a holiday apartment. He spoke almost no English, but communicated through his wife, who spoke limited English, and his son, who was born in the UK. After leaving, he was attended for physiotherapy and occupational therapy (OT) regularly for his injuries. He was attending the OT department as his hands were badly injured. One day he attended the department as usual but found that the doors were being repaired and he would have to enter via the OT kitchen. This caused him to become extremely agitated and distressed and, on discussions with his son, it transpired that he was extremely avoidant of the kitchen at home. The family ran a small take-away restaurant and Chen had often been responsible for most of the cooking before his accident.

The family reported that he was avoiding the kitchen in the family home because of all the traumatic reminders and triggers present, e.g. the cooker, sockets, etc. In view of this it was decided to try and attempt a graded exposure programme with him, starting in the OT kitchen and then at home. However, a meeting (including his wife and son) with his occupational therapist, physiotherapist, keyworker and CBT therapist, to explain and give a rationale of why this would help, soon ran into problems as it became very difficult to explain the principles of the technique to Chen. After much discussion and several failed attempts to explain this, the CBT therapist decided to use the similarities between graded exposure and his regular physiotherapy. His son explained this to Chen and his wife and after some animated discussion between them, they both began smiling and nodding. When asked by the team what had happened, his son said that Chen's wife had told him this was to be 'physiotherapy for his heart' a concept he clearly understood and identified with. Hence the term 'emotional physiotherapy'!

Exposure may involve revisiting the site or scene of the traumatic event. This can be extremely important, if is possible and safe to do so. This allows the person to discriminate 'then' versus 'now' and to develop new meanings about the experience. This should only be attempted at a safe point in therapy and should be therapist-aided, as new meanings may emerge that will need to be addressed in treatment.

To emphasize the importance and value of real-life exposure, we need to revisit Jill's experience after surviving a rail disaster (in Chapter 3). Whilst she found the early counselling helpful, she found it did not address the significant issues of avoidance, which were seriously affecting her ability to work, as well as affecting her social and family life. Her experience of exposure also helped her overcome her many anxieties following her involvement in a rail disaster.

Jill's story (continued)

Later, I changed to a different therapist to focus on rolling back my avoidance behaviours. Initially, I had two sessions of EMDR, which made a difference to anxiety when anticipating rail travel, but I also found the CBT and exposure therapy very beneficial. Under guidance from my therapist I drew up, and followed diligently, a timetable for gradual exposure. It began with building up resilience to driving, through more consistent exposure (which I was also avoiding), then sitting on train platforms, watching trains, building up to repeated train journeys on slow then high-speed trains, over a six-month period.

I also developed mantras/prayers and creative thought patterns to help me cope with my wider range of anxieties. Eighteen months (and about 10 sessions) after beginning the therapy, I feel I am about 75% back to normal with regard to travelling by train and have strategies to help me cope when feeing vulnerable. I am now far more reflective about the train crash and think of it as being more in the past than in the present. I have even recently travelled by air, something I had been dreading!

Exposure in imagination

This involves the patient being asked to relive their traumatic memories, in the first person and present tense, and giving as much detail as possible about the traumatic event and their thoughts, emotions and responses; attention would be paid to specific aspects, e.g. smell, sounds and so on. Often it is possible to construct a hierarchy, using less distressing material first. At the top of the hierarchy are those aspects of the traumatic event that are most upsetting and at the bottom, the least upsetting aspects. Imaginal exposure involves the person working their way up the hierarchy in their imagination, beginning with the least upsetting aspects. The person engages in imagination with their experience until it no longer upsets them. They then move on to the next upsetting aspects and repeat the exercise. At specific points a rewind and hold technique is used, whereby they are asked to concentrate on the worst aspect of the traumatic event, to freeze and hold the image, whilst repeatedly describing in detail all they can remember about this element of the trauma. This is repeated till habituation occurs. The session is audiotaped and they are asked to practice this between sessions, till habituation occurs; a 50–70% reduction in anxiety is desirable for effective reduction in symptoms. As with any exposure therapy, consistency and regular practice is essential. However, the last decade has seen a number of developments in our thinking about the nature of traumatic memories and subsequently more sophisticated approaches based on similar ideas have been developed, such as 'imagery rescripting'.

Imagery rescripting is primarily an experiential technique where the patient is encouraged to think of their problematic and intrusive memories as 'ghosts from the past'. Interestingly, Pierre Janet described examples of 'imagery substitution' in 1889 in his book *L'Automatisme Psychologique*, which mirror the techniques discussed here. The treatment may be roughly explained as follows:

Traumatic events may leave us with distressing images and memories that haunt us and colour our experience of the present. Sometimes these disturbing and upsetting memories are stored with the meanings they had at the time of the event and we think they say a lot about the kind of person we are. Some of these beliefs may be unhelpful, distorted and out of proportion, and no longer valid or true. These memories need to be updated so that they take their proper place in amongst your other memories. The most effective way of doing this is get at the memories by re-experiencing them in your imagination. We can then try and transform them by reflecting on their meanings and using more creative imagery, so they become less distressing.

Common questions during this process may be as follows:

- Is the image you experience based on an actual event?
- What would happen if you allowed the image to continue?
- Can you visualize yourself today having survived the event entering the scene?
- Where are you and what do you see?
- What would the scene look projected onto a cinema screen or seen from a moving train?
- Imagine watching the image on TV, then switching it off, making it smaller, further away, dimmer... freeze the image, make it black and white.

Length of such sessions should be 60–90 minutes and it is important not rush imagery work; several sessions may be needed to deal with one specific memory. There are, therefore, occasions where sessions of CBT may exceed the 8–12 sessions, especially in more complex presentations, as in the case example below using EMDR.

Eye movement desensitization and reprocessing (EMDR)

A technique known as eye movement desensitization and reprocessing (EMDR) is often included as part of CBT. EMDR can be effective in dealing with many trauma symptoms. This is not a 'stand-alone' technique and should be used as part of the course of CBT. EMDR is a relatively new and effective treatment for PTSD, as well as other clinical conditions.

EMDR literally owes its beginnings to a walk in the park. The founder of EMDR, Francine Shapiro, wrote that EMDR was based on a serendipitous discovery made in May 1987. She described that whilst walking through a park, she noticed that she was troubled by some disturbing thoughts, which 'suddenly disappeared'. She also noted that when she tried to recall these thoughts, they were not as disturbing or as valid as they had been previously. She postulated that upsetting thoughts in general had a repetitive quality to them, which only change if the individual does something to stop or change them. However, Shapiro noted that the disturbing thoughts were changing without conscious effort. After paying close attention to this phenomenon, she noticed that during her walk her eyes had moved from side to side and she speculated that this might have been a key factor in her ability to process the disturbing memories. After experimentation with over 70 subjects, she published the first paper on EMDR in 1989.

In essence, EMDR involves pairing memories/disturbing thoughts and the resultant emotions with repeated saccadic (rapid and rhythmic) eye movements, resulting in the desensitization, or reduction in distress caused by the memories. In patients unable to use eye movements, other bi-lateral stimuli, such as hand taps, are used. Hand taps are also used when applying the technique with children, especially younger children, where language may be a problem. A similar pairing of memory and chosen positive cognitions or rational self-statements, with further eye movements (or chosen stumuli), constitutes the reprocessing component. The therapist will ask about changes during the process of EMDR and some of these may be as follows:

- Have you noticed the image change at all?
- Has it become blurred, sharper, more vivid?
- Has it moved further away?
- Has it changed colour?
- What appears different, if anything?
- What bodily changes do you notice, compared to when we started?
- Has your anxiety reduced, remained the same, got worse?

It is often seen as being most useful with what is often described as single-episode trauma, e.g. the road-traffic collision or an assault, but has often been used successfully with longer term accumulative trauma, such as sexual abuse, as illustrated by Sam's story.

Sam's story

Sam is 32 years old. She has eight siblings in total: three male and five female. Six are step-siblings by marriage. Both mother and father had previous marriages with father having four previous children (two male, two female) and mother two (female). Mother and father came together, producing three further children, with Sam being the second to youngest. Sam's eldest sibling is her 45-year-old step-sister.

Sam's father was a paedophile and abused, both physically and sexually, all nine children in varying degrees. Sam's first memory of being abused by her father was around the age of 3 years and the latest at 7 years. Her father also allowed other adult males to sexually abuse Sam. She had an awareness of the sexual abuse to some of her siblings.

Approximately 5 years ago, Sam experienced a crisis and suffered a severe bout of depression. She attended a sexual abuse support group for a year and received one-to-one counselling for a further 6 months. Sam was referred for CBT. She received over 20 sessions of CBT, including EMDR. After the EMDR sessions and when evaluating her therapeutic experience, she reported:

'All I can say is that I have reached a place within myself that I have never been able to before this. I was sceptical and not sure whether it was just

> the right time, the therapy or a combination of both, but EMDR seems to have "shifted" something. I think its strength of belief. It's as though the pain and shit beliefs I've carried all my life about myself have been put down, as though I've finally been able to separate, accept, let go and even, who knows, forgive? Suppose it's just a process really. I've finally been able to make the steps to move on and can't wait to grab the life I now feel is ahead of me.'

EMDR was a controversial technique amongst the psychology and psychotherapy community when first used, but it is now well accepted and used by many therapists working with trauma survivors. The precise mechanism for clinically reported change is as yet unclear and EMDR is still the subject of considerable ongoing research. While there is a growing body of scientific literature on the technique and a number of studies confirm the effectiveness of EMDR in the treatment of PTSD, this does not prove Shapiro's idea that it is because of eye movements. Critics have suggested that EMDR works, not because of anything to do with eye movements but because it involves exposure. However, even if the technique does not work with everyone, it is effective with many trauma survivors.

Medication and drug treatments

Out of the mental health professions, it is only psychiatrists who are permitted to prescribe medication. Some nurses (nurse prescribers) can prescribe medication, but this is rarer in mental health. The NICE guidelines do not recommend medication as a first-line treatment for PTSD. Pharmacological treatments in PTSD sufferers is often considered a critical component of treatment, but it should proceed with a careful and well-thought-out plan, which should be monitored by the therapist, GP and any other mental health professional involved. The most common medication used for PTSD, as an adjunct to psychological therapy, are the selective serotonin reuptake inhibitors (SSRIs). These are usually anti-depressants, some of which are commonly used for PTSD sufferers.

Common concerns of PTSD sufferers about taking medication, such as fears of addiction or of taking medication will be seen as a weakness, should be addressed in early discussions about prescribing options. All patients who are prescribed anti-depressants should be informed, at the time that treatment is started, of potential side-effects and the risk of sudden discontinuation/withdrawal. The onset of discontinuation/withdrawal symptoms is usually within 5 days of stopping the drug. Generally, anti-depressant drugs recommended for use in PTSD should be discontinued over at least a 4-week period, although some people will require longer periods. Written information should be made available, if possible. Most common side-effects are nausea, diarrhoea, abdominal discomfort and sexual dysfunction.

Other therapies

Other therapists are very critical of the idea of PTSD. While these critics would not argue with the fact that people are often considerably distressed following trauma, and experience intrusive thoughts, avoidance, arousal, and so on, what they say is that distress is not an illness. Their point is that we often talk about psychological problems as if they were an illness, but PTSD is not an illness. Instead, these therapists think of therapy as helping the person make sense of their experiences, to confront the existential issues and to make new meanings. The diagnosis of PTSD itself they say can be damaging as, by implying that someone has a condition that needs to be treated, this takes away personal responsibility.

Existential and humanistic therapists can offer people valuable help in working through trauma and what it means to them, and in rebuilding their lives. Like CBT, these are also talking therapies; the difference being that the therapist will be less concerned with assessment, diagnosis and offering a treatment. Rather, the therapist is concerned to understand how you, the client, see things. The therapist wants to understand how it is for you, and to help you make sense of things in your own time and in your own way. The therapist also wants to understand the meaning of the experience for the individual and to help them make sense of it. It is up to the individual to decide what is right for them at the point in their lives they decide to seek help and what their priorities and goals are at that time.

These therapies can be extremely valuable at the right time in a person's life. But as we have seen, avoidance is a big problem with people following trauma and, as such, it may be hard for people to engage with existential and humanistic therapies until they are willing to confront their experiences. Some of the treatments for PTSD can therefore be useful to pave the way for these other therapies, which help some people to want to explore deeper meanings of their experiences. For many, trauma-focused CBT will be effective in not only dealing with PTSD symptoms, but also with issues of guilt and shame. As we will see in Chapter 8, trauma can often be a turning point in people's lives and, as such, good therapists will help individuals to find meaning and renegotiate their priorities in light of their traumatic experience whatever therapy they practice.

The impact of litigation on the course of treatment and recovery

One issue that often affects trauma survivors is the issue of litigation, especially following road-traffic collisions and industrial injury. There have also been many high-profile compensation cases concerning veterans and individuals who have developed a medical condition or suffered an injury or loss as a result of medical negligence. While it is appropriate in many cases for people to seek compensation for psychological suffering, this can be problematic in its own right. It is often the case that medico-legal process, which can be protracted and complicated, serve's to prolong people's distress. It is the exception rather than the rule that individual's 'invent' their symptoms and are driven by the anticipated financial rewards.

Most medico-legal cases seen by the vast majority of psychologists, psychotherapists, psychiatrists and other mental health professionals, are genuine. If, for example, anyone is involved in a road-traffic collision or industrial accident that was caused by someone else and liability is admitted, then the individual is legitimately entitled to compensation through the other party's insurance. This can be for either physical or psychiatric injury. The amount of compensation is calculated by reference to a variety of factors, e.g. loss of earnings, the nature of damage or injury, the impact on social and occupational functioning, costs of treatments for physical or psychological care. Claimants are advised as to the amount they may be entitled to by their legal representatives, they *do not*, contrary to popular belief, decide upon the amount themselves. There is also little or no evidence for what is known as 'compensation neuroses'. This is when someone is seen to be exaggerating or prolonging their symptoms and the impact this has on their lives in order to gain a greater financial settlement. Previous studies of victims of road-traffic collisions or accidental injury have shown that symptoms do not disappear or improve when the legal process has come to an end. Of course there are always individual examples that could be cited to the contrary, but these would be the exception rather than the rule.

At the time of writing, a documentary has been aired on prime-time television entitled the 'Trauma Industry', focusing on compensation issues and subsequently the legitimacy, and possible overuse, of the PTSD diagnosis. The programme grossly misrepresented the plight of those who have suffered a traumatic experience through the fault or negligence of others. It was overly simplistic and failed to convey the complexities and intricacies that bedevil those going through the process of litigation. The medico-legal process can be a difficult and unpleasant experience that many individuals persevere with, not because they want financial rewards, but because they wish justice to be done. Before embarking on a course of action for medico-legal compensation, it is worth considering the following:

- The solicitor for the claimant usually obtains a medical report in the first instance, prior to the issue of any court proceedings, after agreeing the identity of the expert to be instructed with the other party's insurers or solicitor. However, if after considering the report the other party is unhappy with the findings in the report, then they may seek to obtain their own expert's report. For instance, the other party may seek to argue that pre-existing vulnerabilities are the prime cause of distress, rather than any psychiatric or psychological injury resulting from the accident. This can make the Claimant feel that their honesty is being questioned in some way.

- The person often has to attend many appointments with what are known as 'expert witnesses'. These are professional experts in their field in either physical medicine or mental health, e.g. orthopaedics, psychiatry, psychology or other specialty.

- These appointments invariably involve travel, sometimes over long distances if the expert is not local. This in itself can be stressful, because it may involve the individual (or their partner or relative) having time off from work and it may in itself be financially costly.

- The assessments often, if not always, involve repeated telling of the story, sometimes in great detail.

- Under the court rules the solicitors for each party can agree to appoint what is known as a joint expert, which means that both parties agree to be bound by the single expert's opinion however favourable or unfavourable that may be. This has the benefit of removing the need for a person to see more than one expert in each speciality but is not always appropriate in all cases.

- Under the law the burden is on the injured party to prove fault, rather than the other party proving they are not at fault, which some people feel is unfair. This can enhance the sense of injustice they already feel.

- In cases where the other party denies any liability for the claimant's claim, court proceedings often have to be issued in order to progress matters and ultimately the claimant may have to appear in court to give evidence in person. This is often a source of serious concern to an individual, which can compound their other problems. However, the majority of claims are settled out of court.

- Reports often take time to produce and sometimes many weeks may elapse before the report is produced. However, it is the ethical responsibility of the expert to produce the report as soon as possible in order not to delay the process. This inevitably involves more delays as legal teams then have to consider what action needs to be taken in their client's best interest and the financial implications. Medico-legal reports should ideally be produced as soon as possible after the assessment, but a reasonable time-frame should be within two to three weeks of the assessment date.

- If recommendations for treatment are made, then applications for funding have to be made in order to facilitate that, as most of these treatments, whilst available under the NHS, may involve long waiting-lists and therefore private treatment is often sought.

- The majority of compensation payments are not large. Sums of six or seven figures are rare but are more likely to be in the tens of thousands. Large compensation payments are usually made when there is a loss of life, limb or the person needs long-term treatment or care, e.g. following a head or spinal injury.

- Compensation for criminal injuries are most often made through the Criminal Injuries Compensation Authority and again, these sums are not vast and are awarded on a tariff system for injuries, which many victims often see as unfair. However, there is an appeals process in place for those who contest their awards.

- Any payments made prior to a final settlement, known as 'interim payments', e.g. for the cost of travel, subsistence, any preliminary treatments, investigations and assessments, are deducted from the final settlement to avoid 'double recovery' under the law, something many are not aware of, as it is often not made explicit. Therefore these issues should be discussed with the legal representative.

It must be noted that the laws surrounding compensation for psychiatric injury will differ between countries and there also differences in the UK between Scottish and English law. This will also differ in other countries.

Conclusion

Therapeutic approaches, such as CBT, including techniques like EMDR, have been demonstrated to be effective with PTSD sufferers. These approaches work by facilitating a constructive engagement with their fears, avoidances and shattered assumptions about themselves, others and the world, enabling survivors to develop new meanings and make sense of their experience. Other therapies can also be helpful, such as existential and humanistic therapies, in providing an opportunity for people to confront any existential issues they may be struggling with. These forms of therapy are less active and directive in nature. They may often be helpful to those people who want to explore issues and experiences that they feel have been brought to the fore as a direct or indirect result of the traumatic event. It must be emphasized that different therapies will suit different people and at different times in their lives. The individual needs to decide what is best suited to their circumstances, needs and goals at the time they seek help.

6

Medically related trauma

Key points

- Post-traumatic symptoms and post-traumatic stress disorder (PTSD) often present following medical procedures and illnesses.

- Research has shown that post-traumatic stress can result from accidental injury, burn trauma, cancer and other life-threatening conditions.

- Negative experiences of childbirth can also lead to post-traumatic symptoms and PTSD.

- Medically related trauma is different from other traumatic events because it can be seen as 'continuous traumatic stress' rather than 'post', because of ongoing complications, repeated surgery and other invasive procedures.

The prevalence of trauma and PTSD in medical settings

Having considered the epidemiology and prevalence surrounding post-traumatic stress in a wider context, we will now focus on the specific prevalence of trauma and PTSD in the above areas. In addition, PTSD symptoms have also been described after medical illness and treatment, e.g. cardiac arrest survivors, general surgical units, in stroke patients, following a diagnosis of breast cancer and after childbirth. This chapter will present an overview of some of the likely and perhaps less obvious, areas where post-traumatic stress may present, either on its own or as part of a broader picture of psychological distress.

In this chapter we will also look at the impact of physical injuries following industrial accidents and road-traffic collisions. There will also be some suggestions as to how some longer term psychological difficulties may be avoided by adopting some relatively simple strategies at an early stage.

Modern medicine often uses invasive procedures, for which most individuals have little real preparation or understanding. Health professionals are not infallible, and mistakes and accidents unfortunately can, and do, occur during medical procedures. A complication occurring during a procedure, or a medical accident, can have profound effects upon the individual. In addition to the

Table 6.1 Prevalence rates of PTSD in relation to different events in medical settings

Burn injury	7–45%
Child's life-threatening illness	10%
Child's unexpected death	45%
Myocardial Infarction	9%
Obstetric/gynaecological procedures	1.7–6%
Road-traffic accidents	10–46%
Stroke	9.8%
Sudden death of a 'loved one' (adult)	14%

trauma and shock that a complication or error has caused, the individual also has to contend with the fact that the very people who they felt were there to help them, have played a role in their distress. This can give rise to feelings of helplessness and uncontrollability, as well as a future loss of trust in health professionals, distrust of future diagnosis and advice, and fear of future treatments. Some researchers have concluded that post-traumatic stress is prolonged after medical events, presumably due in part to the uncontrollability of the situation, for the individual affected.

Fay's story

Fay 47, underwent a planned admission to a surgical ward to undergo a hysterectomy. She had been an inpatient previously, during which she found all of the staff she encountered to be helpful and supportive, and was left with a positive view of 'hospitals'. Consequently she had a positive outlook prior to her admission for a hysterectomy. Unfortunately, during the operation problems occurred resulting in her being admitted to an intensive care unit (ICU) for six days, following which she developed an infection requiring a total hospital stay in excess of three weeks. Fay felt that staff on the ward that she went to from ICU treated her unsympathetically, in that she believed that the staff thought she was 'over-reacting' about the amount of pain and discomfort she was experiencing. Her symptoms included: flashbacks, nightmares, avoidance of hospitals (and of all media triggers concerning medical matters), a sense of foreshortened future (feelings that her life may somehow be cut short) and high level of irritability/anger.

Road-traffic collisions

The most common presentation in trauma and orthopaedic units will be those arising from a variety of accidental injuries, ranging from road-traffic collisions (RTCs) to industrial accidents. In 2007, 646 pedestrians were killed in road accidents in Great Britain. The total number of deaths in road-accident collisions fell by 7% to to 2,946 in 2007 from 3,172 in 2006. However, the number of fatalities has remained fairly constant over the last ten years. Nearly half (49%) of people killed in road accidents were car users in 2007. Pedal cyclists and motor cyclists represented 5 and 20% of those killed, respectively. The total number of road casualties of all severities was approximately 280,000 in 2007. The range of RTC survivors includes pedestrians, motorcyclists and cyclists. However, the research literature on RTCs has tended to focus on motor vehicle accidents *per se*. The rates for PTSD following RTCs vary from 11% to 46%. In a study of a consecutive series of 188 RTC victims, a quarter described long-term psychiatric consequences of three overlapping types:

- mood disorder;
- post-traumatic stress disorder;
- phobic anxiety about travel.

In addition, a fifth of people complained of persistent and disabling anxiety. One-fifth of the sample with major or minor injuries experienced severe initial distress, characterized by altered mood and horrific memories. Nineteen of the sample (11%) met the criteria for PTSD at one year.

Michaela's story

Michaela is a 28-year-old professional woman who was admitted following a serious RTC and has suffered severe multiple injuries. She had stopped on the motorway to help at an accident. She saw another driver running towards her waving at her to stop and help. As she stopped on the hard shoulder and was preparing to get out of out of the car, her car and the other driver were hit by a lorry travelling at speed, which could not stop in time. The other man was killed instantly and she was trapped in the car and had to be cut out by the emergency services. After three weeks in hospital, she was having tearful episodes, experiencing problems sleeping (unrelated to pain), was low in mood and expressing feelings of guilt at having survived when someone else had died. When originally offered help by the ward staff, she had declined, but then later requested to be seen.

She was given the opportunity to discuss the circumstances of the accident (which she had previously not done in any depth for fear of upsetting her relatives), her thoughts and emotional reactions at the time, her current difficulties and reactions, e.g. her guilt feelings. She also expressed her anxieties about what she had been told by friends and relatives about the accident, as she had a poor memory of events. As a consequence, she had formed her own narrative based on what she'd been told, thus she had 'reconstructed' memories, some of which were inaccurate, as confirmed by the police and eyewitnesses. The issue of 'reconstructed memory' was discussed in some depth and she was able to develop a more accurate narrative, which helped her deal with the guilt she had been feeling over the death of the other driver. She was provided with education, advice and guidance, as described above, and encouraged to ask questions about her reactions and responses. Her reactions were normalized in the context of her experience. She was later seen once on the ward for follow-up and then in the outpatient department. Six months later, she was making a good recovery with no psychological ill effects. She reported that the early session and the follow-up had helped make sense of her feelings and reactions at the time and in the subsequent days and weeks.

Coping with the effects of traumatic injury

Physical injury following accidents, such as road-traffic collisions, can be classed as one of the 'complicating' factors that we looked at earlier. The reason for this is that such injuries, often regardless of their magnitude, can impact upon psychological recovery. This often happens because of the repeated visits to hospital for surgery, physiotherapy and other treatments. For example, following a burn trauma, this can mean repeated appointments for surgery for skin-grafting and correction of previous surgery. It can also impact upon work and employment prospects and inevitably affect levels of social and leisure activity. Previously, avoidance following traumatic events has been noted to be common but lead to problems in the longer term if not monitored and dealt with gradually and systematically over time. However, with individuals who have suffered a physical injury, there is often an 'enforced avoidance' because of practical reasons, which can lead to further problems later. For example, the person may have had a severe leg injury, which would inhibit their levels of physical activity and mobility and, consequently, they would have to forego many activities they would previously have undertaken, for the simple reason they are physically unable to carry them out. This 'enforced avoidance' may often lead to a gradual reduction of social contact and, therefore, a reduction of social support, leading to the development of symptoms, such as mental and behavioural avoidance and the reduction of confidence, self-esteem and mood. This then feeds back into the cycle of a loss of routine and inactivity, and a reduction of social contact, and eventually becomes a very difficult pattern to break. There are some useful strategies in the wake of being exposed to a traumatic injury, and by this we mean injuries that have been sustained in circumstances that are sudden, unexpected, often violent and sometimes life-threatening, such as road-traffic collisions, industrial accidents, workplace violence and transportation accidents, which may involve multiple fractures, serious lacerations and amputations.

Some useful strategies are as follows:

- Try to establish a routine as soon as possible—when you get home from hospital, try and consider ways in which you can be active, however small at first, during the day and through the week.

- Draw up an activity schedule for each week and, if necessary, break each day into one-hour time slots.

- Don't be over-ambitious at the start, pace yourself; a little is better than too much—don't set yourself up to fail.

- Try not to sleep during the day—this can be difficult but planning activities would help.

- Try and keep a sleep diary, ask others to help you with this, noting your sleep patterns, wherever possible.

- With regard to activity—think of things you used to like doing but are not able to do now—is it possible to try some of these activities in a small way given your limitations?

- Think of things you have perhaps always wanted to do or learn about but have never had the time to try—this might be a good opportunity to ask somebody to get you information from the library or other sources in order to try and acquire new knowledge or perhaps a skill, if that is possible.

- Try and incorporate the activities into a schedule for the week.

- Be practical, don't overdo it. Start with 10–15-minute periods—don't attempt activities for unreasonably long periods, e.g. an hour or more. You may find you become tired quite soon, have to give up the activity and then either blame yourself or find it difficult to return and continue where you left off.

- Try to be consistent.

- Remember!! It is better to do something for a brief period of time than nothing at all.

- As seen before, activity has a positive effect on mood over time.

Burn trauma

Within the last decade there has been an emerging interest in the complex nature of post-traumatic symptoms and PTSD following burn injury. There is evidence that post-traumatic symptoms and PTSD are not uncommon in burn survivors. In the UK, about 500 deaths per year occur as a result of injury by fire, and over 28,000 suffer serious injuries. In the USA, it is estimated that approximately 1% annually of the population sustains burns, i.e. approximately 300,000 people, of whom 7000 die. It would be hardly surprising if burn injury, which is a painful, frightening and extraordinary traumatic event, precipitated post-traumatic symptoms in some burns survivors. Other risk and vulnerability factors found to be important were age, social class and whether individuals lived on their own or with large family, pointing to the importance again of social support. There is also no clear relationship between where the injury occurs on the body and the frequency and severity of psychological side-effects.

Research conducted with some of the most severely physically damaged survivors of the King's Cross fire in 1987, showed that many were troubled by nightmares (invariably involving flames); all described a heightened sense of vigilance in everyday situations, e.g. crossing the road. They also experienced an intense sense of the frailty of human life and an expectation of further disasters. Many reported flashbacks, disturbed sleep, avoidance of common activities and emotional difficulties on the anniversary of the disaster—all symptoms characteristic of PTSD.

The lesson to be learned here is, as the authors of the study concluded, that:

> ...early psychological contact is vital for the emotional and physical well-being of the patient in the early stages of recovery.

The development of PTSD in children post-burn has also been studied. Researchers have found that when compared with other clinical samples of children, children who suffered burn trauma had especially high levels of psychiatric disturbance, including PTSD. Some believe that the burn treatment itself becomes a traumatic event, and that, for some children, the longer hospitalization is extended, with the daily cycle of dressing changes and physiotherapy, the more regressed and withdrawn they become.

Jane and Robert's story

Jane, 29, and her 2-year-old son Robert were the survivors of an explosion that occurred in the family home. The accident occurred a few days before Christmas. Jane was also three months pregnant at the time. The boiler exploded, virtually demolishing the living room and causing severe damage estimated at £12,000.

Robert was seriously injured, suffering a depressed fracture of the frontal lobe of the brain and 12% burns, which required grafting; the areas of most concern being his right forehead (the eyebrow being missing) and the right side of his torso. Jane sustained burns to both legs, mostly superficial. She also received a head injury, sustained when she was hit by flying debris. Both mother and son were taken to the local A&E department and then admitted to the burns unit. Her unborn child was unharmed.

After the accident, she suffered from depression and also experienced a variety of symptoms, which met the diagnostic criteria for PTSD. She was unable to discuss her son's injuries (which were severe) or her own. She would avoid television programmes, magazines or newspaper articles containing material that reminded her of the accident. She was experiencing panic attacks, bouts of irritability and exhibiting obsessional behaviour, resulting in frequent checking of electrical appliances, such as the gas fire and the cooker.

Her relationship with her husband was also under considerable strain and she found that she was becoming overprotective and over-concerned with her son's welfare, the latter inevitably having implications for his future psychological development and well-being. Jane was unable to discuss the accident with anybody she might meet on a casual or social basis; she would become extremely distressed and withdraw from the situation. Jane was also experiencing bouts of anxiety triggered by the continuing treatment Robert required because of his injuries. Jane also had marked concern about Robert's ability to integrate with other children, owing to the cosmetic nature of his injuries, and worried lest this caused problems at school and in later life; to some extent, her concerns were not without substance.

Jane also experienced feelings of guilt and anger about the incident and her part in Robert's aftercare. She felt that she could have done more at the time of the accident to help to remove him from the scene of the explosion. She recalled that at the time of the accident, she made every attempt to try to reach her son, but was so bewildered, shocked and frightened that she could not locate him, as the room was in darkness and she was also handicapped by her own injuries. Consequently, she made for the nearest chink of light and stumbled free to get help. She began to see this as an act of selfishness rather than the only course of action open to her at the time.

Jane received 12 sessions of CBT and was able to make a good recovery, develop new perspectives and coping strategies. Her recovery had a positive effect on Robert who was able to integrate well with other children, often being overheard by teachers at school discussing his experiences, both of the accident and at hospital with the other children in a positive way.

> Even if you are badly hurt, the doctors and nurses at the hospital are great! They can make things better most of the time… and they have loads of great DVDS!'

PTSD resulting from obstetric trauma

Studies from various countries suggest a prevalence of between 0 and 7% of women fulfilling diagnostic criteria for PTSD at some point after giving birth. Prevalence rates are higher in at-risk groups, such as women who have a premature or stillbirth, with reports of up to 26%. Cross-cultural comparison of prevalence rates suggests similar prevalence in Europe (i.e. Sweden, Italy, UK and The Netherlands), the USA and Australia.

The available evidence seems to suggest that the prevalence of PTSD in women after birth in developed countries is approximately 1–2%.

In a review of 500 women's experiences of obstetric and gynaecological procedures, over a 100 described their experiences as being 'very distressing' or 'terrifying'. Of these women, at follow-up, 30 of them met the criteria for PTSD. These women identified that they experienced feelings of powerlessness during the procedure, a lack of information as to the procedures taking place, the experience of physical pain and a perceived 'unsympathetic' attitude on the part of the staff.

Research has described PTSD resulting from obstetric trauma, where the labour was medically complicated, painful, prolonged and threatening to the life of the mother and the baby. Another study into childbirth experiences in Sweden found post-traumatic stress reactions after emergency Caesarean sections. Of 25 women were interviewed a few days and a few months after emergency section, 19 had experienced their delivery as a traumatic event but, at after 2 months, none of the women met the criteria of PTSD. However, 13 women had various forms of post-traumatic stress reactions and some of these had high levels of intrusive thoughts.

Jan's story

Jan was a 31-year-old mother of two who was having her third child. She began having contractions earlier than anticipated, which eventually resulted in her being taken to hospital. As she was staying with friends for the weekend, in another city, she was taken to a hospital she did not know. She developed unexpected complications and, during delivery in the labour suite, she suffered a significant loss of blood. She recalled a lot of doctors and midwives being present, a lot of noise and activity, and then, as she was drifting in and out of consciousness, she heard a male voice saying, 'I think we are losing her...'—she wasn't sure if this meant her or the baby, as both she and her partner knew that it was a girl. Soon after she lost consciousness and when she woke in the antenatal unit the following day, she felt disorientated, her surroundings felt strange and unreal and she was convinced that she had died. She gradually realized this wasn't the case when she saw her daughter beside her.

Nevertheless, the experience left her with marked post-traumatic reactions, which later developed into significant symptoms of PTSD. She did not understand what was happening to her and why she was feeling the way she was. This very much echoes Laura's story earlier. As is often usual, she began to avoid thinking and talking about her experience, which subsequently led to other avoidances, such as crossing the street when she saw a mother and baby, reading newspaper or magazine articles about pregnancy and childbirth, and switching off the TV or changing channels if she saw programmes that had a resonance to her experience.

Conclusion

The experience of traumatic events often results in the shattering of basic assumptions that the victims hold about themselves, others and the world. It is common for this to occur after a traumatic injury or traumatic experiences resulting from medical procedures. There are three basic assumptions about the self, others and the world that are commonly shared by most people. We may not be aware of these, but they are often related to the following:

◆ the belief in personal invulnerability, i.e. nothing is going to happen to us;
◆ the perception of the world as meaningful and comprehensible, i.e. generally there is a predictability to our lives;
◆ the view of self and others in a positive light.

Therefore, the assessment of attribution and meaning is vital in understanding an individual's reactions following traumatic events. Traumatic events have the potential to shatter these basic assumptions. The relevance of shattered assumptions and the significance of anger are worth bearing in mind. Anger is a common emotional reaction in victims of trauma. However, it can also prove to be an extremely debilitating emotion. It often focuses on the lack of concern or apology from those believed to be responsible and the lack of recognition of the suffering and disability caused.

Some of this distress can be diffused by a simple, straightforward explanation of their difficulties; to be told that they are responding in a normal way to a distressing experience, and what course their symptoms may take, i.e. that the majority of individuals return to normal emotional functioning within a few days/weeks.

7

Cultural responses to trauma

Key points

- Cultural responses to trauma and loss vary depending on age, cultural and ethnic differences and gender.

- Within different cultures, PTSD may not always appear be appropriate as a diagnosis, but often the symptoms overall tend to fit a consistent picture.

- It is possible to adapt different therapies to work with refugees and survivors of torture, but this needs to be considered alongside other community-based approaches.

- Humanitarian aid agencies are developing psycho-social programmes to cater to the needs of individuals, families and communities affected by complex emergencies, such as natural disasters and civil conflict.

- Psycho-social programmes are designed to promote and enhance the natural resilience of populations affected by complex emergencies.

Introduction

Cultural responses to traumatic events are often complex, and psychological reactions will vary depending on age, cultural and ethnic differences and gender. In addition, the notion of psychotherapy or counselling will often be an alien concept as access to 'talking therapies' are rare and many cultures would turn to traditional healers. However, this will be covered later in the chapter. The awareness of the impact of traumatic events on different cultures and societies has become widespread in an age where advances in communication technologies mean that the human costs following conflict, disasters and other emergencies are brought into our lives, not only through the media of television but also through readily available access to the internet. It is beyond the scope of this book to examine cultural responses in significant depth, but the intention here is to give an overview of cultural factors that may influence and affect individuals and communities experience of traumatic events.

Firstly, the impact of trauma on refugees will be discussed and then there will be an overview of what humanitarian aid organizations are currently doing to address the needs of populations affected by conflict, disaster and what are often described as 'complex emergencies'. These are situations where one humanitarian disaster or catastrophe is affected by another, such as in Sri Lanka and Aceh in Indonesia, where the impact of the Tsunami and relief efforts were complicated by many years of civil conflict in the affected areas.

The concept of psychological trauma and cultural differences across cultures

Across cultures, people differ in what they believe and understand about life and death, what they feel, what elicits those feelings, the perceived implications of those feelings, their expression and appropriateness of certain feelings and strategies for dealing with feelings that cannot be directly expressed. A cross-cultural perspective demonstrates the variety, for example, in people's responses to death and dying, and the process of mourning. Rather than being process-orientated, mourning is seen as an adaptive response to specific task demands arising from loss that must be dealt with regardless of individual, culture or historical era. Stroebe (1992) challenged the belief in the importance of 'grief work' for adjustment to bereavement. She examined claims made in theoretical formulations and principles of grief counselling and therapy concerning the necessity of working through loss. Grief reactions are also patterned by the culture, formed by one's society's belief systems and expectations, values and norms for relationships and bonds. This will influence both expression and duration of grief reactions across different cultural settings. In essence, sensitivity to the culturally appropriate needs for ritual, in responding to grief and providing for privacy and personal needs, are paramount.

Research on post-traumatic reactions in non-Western groups has mostly been conducted in Western Europe and the United States to meet the needs of refugees from developing countries. Differences in the prevalence of PTSD across ethnic and cultural groups have been reported. However, there are several problematic issues related to cross-cultural trauma research. One of the reasons for discrepancies in cross-cultural studies is that Western diagnostic criteria are not always applicable in non-Western cultures and the diagnosis of PTSD has been controversial.

For example, a recent study on Tibetan refugees in India, demonstrated that in this population the destruction of religious symbols was a major stressor. If culturally defined stressors are not heeded, the amount of stress experienced would be evaluated lower than it actually was. The same group of workers also noted that some symptoms common to trauma survivors, such as guilt, were displayed far less than would be expected, explained by the fact that the word 'guilt' does not even have a Tibetan equivalent. A further illustration can be seen in the above study within a religious context. Buddhism implies that 'hopelessness lies in the nature of the world'. The acknowledgement of the all-pervasive presence of suffering in the world is almost 'endorsed' by Buddhism. A 'non-disorder' frame of reference for 'depressive' symptoms is therefore present within Buddhist cultures. A recent study that attempted to assess PTSD in a radically non-Western culture, that of Kalahari Bushmen, found that the results compared closely with PTSD assessments in other non-Western societies.

There have been a number of studies conducted with survivors of torture and political violence, which have shown that the most common symptoms displayed across the cultures sampled, were those associated with the diagnoses of depression, anxiety disorders and post-traumatic stress disorder (PTSD). They manifest themselves in different ways within cultures, but the symptoms tend to fit the general diagnostic criteria for the disorders mentioned above. Some individuals will also have suffered multiple losses, in addition to their torture experiences.

Definition of torture

In 1984, the United Nations, in the Convention against Torture and Other Cruel, Inhuman or Degrading Treatment or Punishment, adopted the following definition:

For the purpose of this Convention, the term 'torture' means any act by which severe pain or suffering, whether physical or mental, is intentionally inflicted on a person for such purpose as obtaining from him or a third person information or a confession, punishing him for an act he or a third person has committed, or is suspected of having committed, or intimidating or coercing him or a third person, or for any reason based on discrimination of any kind, when such pain or suffering is inflicted by, or at the instigation of, or with the consent or acquiescence of, a public official or other person acting in an official capacity. It does not include pain or suffering arising only from, inherent in or incidental to lawful sanctions.

This definition was restricted to apply only to nations and to government-sponsored torture. It did not include cases of countries where torture, such as mutilation or whipping, are practices of lawful punishment, nor did it include cases of torture practiced by gangs or hate groups. In 1986, the WHO working group introduced the concept of Organized Violence, which was defined as:

The inter-human infliction of significant, avoidable pain and suffering by an organized group according to a declared or implied strategy and/or system of ideas and attitudes. It comprises any violent action that is unacceptable by general human standards, and relates to the victim's feelings. Organized violence includes 'torture, cruel inhuman or degrading treatment or punishment' as in Article 5 of the United Nations

Universal Declaration of Human Rights (1948). Imprisonment without trial, mock executions, hostage-taking, or any other form of violent deprivation of liberty, also falls under the heading of organized violence.

Torture is a complex trauma that often occurs within the context of widespread persecution and human rights violations. Furthermore, the nature of modern armed conflict is such that whole populations are at risk of suffering extensive trauma, losses, injustices and displacement. The estimates of the numbers of asylum seekers who have been victims of torture or organized violence vary considerably, depending on their country of origin and definitions used. The UNHCR estimated:

- In 2007, the total number of refugees, asylum seekers and others of concern numbered 19.2 million.
- 20.6 million people are 'of concern'—*1 out of every 300 people on earth.*
- There are 25–30 million internally displaced people (IDP) worldwide.
- Women and children make up three-quarters of the estimated figure of the 20.6 million people of concern.
- The United Nations High Commission for Refugees (UNHCR) is caring for approximately 6,000,000 IDP worldwide.

Assessment of trauma across cultures

The massive trauma experienced by refugees and torture victims raises ethical and clinical questions about the potential negative impact upon them of using checklists or questionnaires, as have previously described. Secondly, the diverse ethno-cultural and political backgrounds require assessment questionnaires sensitive to a wide range of traumatic events and experiences. For example, the traumatic experiences of Chilean political prisoners were dramatically different to those of Indo-Chinese refugees. Finally, while specific symptoms have been clearly linked to the trauma of torture, the DSM-IV criterion for PTSD has not been established as a valid disease construct in non-Western cultures. Cross-national comparisons by the World Health Organization (WHO) suggest that, despite core features of major depression, each culture has its own specific symptoms. PTSD criteria may reveal a similar pattern across cultures; however, a central universal core of PTSD remains to be established. There are issues concerning the definition and nature of traumatic stressors in different cultures. These are often different depending on the cultural settings. Therefore, a standardized checklist could under- or over-estimate the prevalence of traumatic stressors, if the list was not sensitive to the cultural values of the population studied.

Nevertheless, there have been a number of studies conducted with disaster survivors, refugees, survivors of torture and political violence, which used the most culturally appropriate assessment methods available. It would appear that the most common symptoms displayed across the cultures sampled in the above studies, were those associated with the diagnoses of depression, anxiety and PTSD. They manifest themselves in different ways within cultures, but the symptoms tend to fit the general diagnostic criteria for the disorders mentioned above. In recent years there have also been studies that have attempted to address the issue of assessment and the use of culturally sensitive questionnaires with some degree of success.

Recently, critics of the concept of PTSD as applied to non-Western settings have also argued that there is no evidence that mental health problems are higher in populations exposed to conflict and other complex emergencies, citing Northern Ireland as one such example. Critics further suggest that over the last 30 years of civil conflict there has been little evidence of significant impact on referral rates to mental health services. However, a recent published community survey to assess the effects of the civil unrest (the Troubles as they have come to be known) on the general population concluded that exposure to the Troubles has resulted in a significant and independent detrimental effect on the mental health of the population in Northern Ireland. Within the context of the Northern Ireland Troubles we are drawn to the observations of Arlene Healy, Consultant Family Therapist and Head of the Family Trauma Centre in Belfast who has written eloquently about the 'context of silence' in Northern Ireland. When discussing her work with children and families affected by the troubles she provides an explanation for the perceived lack of mental health problems within the population of the province.

She discusses the context of silence that has existed for almost thirty years. Silence from those involved and from social services; silence within higher education establishments and those involved in the education and training of health and social care professionals; the silence amongst those planning health and social care provision in the province.

She has argued that finding a language adequately explaining the impact of trauma on families was difficult because of the vacuum of silence that surrounded decades of violence in which a language to discuss such traumatic events failed to develop. By 1994, the peace process had gained momentum, a sense of hope was growing—it began to be easier to discuss the impact of the troubles. Society in Northern Ireland had also reflected this change through the media and in literature, which reflected this newly found sense of hope. The establishment of a Victims Commission in 1998, following the publication of the Bloomfield report, led to the setting up of a Family Trauma Centre in 1999, a province-wide service. Furthermore, there has been the establishment of Trauma Advisory Panels in Northern Ireland—a clear acceptance that the mental health needs of the population in relation to their traumatic experiences warrant addressing. In addition, the Cost of the Troubles Study, concluded that 30% of those who participated in and had been exposed to violence associated with the troubles had needs approximating to post-traumatic stress disorder and related conditions. These factors were further supported in a recent review of mental health and learning disability in Northern Ireland, which supported the view that psychological trauma, had not been sufficiently addressed as a specific health issue.

Factors affecting asylum seekers and refugees

Health and mental health practitioners are accustomed to seeing culturally diverse populations in their regular practice. Inevitably, many will be refugees who are survivors of torture and organized violence. Whilst not all will experience such extremes of traumatic events, these particular individuals often present to therapists with complex psychotherapeutic challenges. For many there will be normal and understandable problems of adjustment to a new culture and society, combined with the practical problems presented by the host country's asylum processes and procedures. There will be no attempt to describe these laws and processes here, as they vary considerably from country to country and are often subject to frequent changes influenced by national priorities and international events. Universally, those fleeing wars, religious or ethnic persecution were once referred to collectively as refugees. However over the last decade, the term 'asylum seeker' has been adopted and used by almost all EU countries. Essentially, this means the same thing in these countries, that is those seeking a safe haven are given the status of 'asylum seekers' until their cases have been heard and they are given the right to stay in the country, whereby they are then given 'refugee' status and usually able to access rights and benefits available to citizens of the host country. One common factor pertinent to all asylum seekers is the inability to seek or obtain paid employment before they are granted refugee status. This inevitably has significant implications for the mental health of individuals and families, as it is well known that access to employment has a positive impact on mental health and well-being. There is also great variability in other areas, such as access to housing, healthcare, legal aid, interpreters and other resources to improve the quality of their lives.

Where asylum seekers and refugees have been welcomed and offered opportunities to develop their potential and capacities, participate actively in the affairs of the host country, they often overcome major adversities from their past. On the other hand, where they are marginalized, victimized and held back, they tend to become enmeshed in stereotypical roles that reinforce negative beliefs and values, leading to further persecution and repression. After periods of upheaval, most individuals and communities become proactive in efforts to re-establish their equilibrium and take steps to achieve recovery and promote well-being. Common problems experienced by those seeking asylum and refugees are:

◆ A loss of identity.

◆ Being scapegoated by host society, often leading to isolation, hostility, violence, racism.

- Being dependant on state benefits to survive.
- Not having adequate access to health and social care benefits.
- Experiencing high levels of psychosomatic complaints, i.e. presenting with physical problems often masking psychological difficulties.
- Problems of adjustment to the host society and local community.
- Depression.
- Anxiety, guilt and shame.
- Symptoms of post-traumatic stress and PTSD.

By attempting to define and establish more clearly the links between types of trauma, cultural, mental and social mechanisms and structures that influence these experiences, and the ongoing post-traumatic social environment, it may be possible to intervene early with those refugees at greatest risk of persisting psychological and social disability. It will be inevitable that refugees will often only respond to therapists who adopt an unambiguous position in supporting their human rights—an important ethical and practical consideration.

Issues relating to treatment

It is vital to establish a good rapport with the patient at the outset. An understanding of the social, cultural and political landscape of the torture survivor is important. Giving the message that the therapist has taken time to try to understand and make sense of the circumstances that lead them to seek asylum is key to establishing a good rapport and relationship. It is also useful to try and speak a few simple words in the patient's own language, if possible. A simple greeting or welcoming phrase in the patient's own language can make a significant difference. The role of the interpreter is crucial. In many cases, the only qualification the interpreter has is the ability to speak another language. They will often have little, if any, training in mental health issues. Guidelines for therapists and interpreters are given in more detail below.

Close collaboration is recommended with other services, such as physiotherapy, which can often assist in dealing with the numerous physical problems manifested by torture survivors, such as muscular skeletal problems and the effects of other physical injuries. Linking and liaising with community resources at an early stage is vital in trying to bridge the divide between the voluntary and statutory services. It is also useful to have information on the survivors' host country and the context of their experience. The development of a 'Country File' can be a useful resource, with information being gleaned from a variety of websites (see Appendix 3). This can hold updates on the country of origin, together with previous and current political developments, historical and geographical information, human rights violations and related information. Knowledge and awareness of some of these issues can have a significant positive impact on the establishment of the relationship and rapport, between the practitioner and torture survivor. Medication also has a place in the range of therapeutic options found effective in helping survivors. There are also clear indications that selective anti-depressants can show benefits, if used appropriately, in specific cases.

It is beyond the scope of this chapter to provide details of which therapies are the most effective, but many different approaches have been used and often therapists may use a combination of approaches and strategies. Recently case reports have been published demonstrating that CBT can be useful with survivors of torture. Cognitive behavioral interventions also involve encouraging survivors to think that their behavior under torture was a normal human response necessary for survival; that torture is designed to induce total loss of control and helplessness, which might explain why they behaved the way they did. Torture survivors also need to establish new values and assumptions about themselves, others and the world that enable the development of trust, meaning and more functional behaviors. However, therapy should not be seen as an activity that happens in isolation. Another extremely important aspect of treatment is the integration of the patient into the community. This involves the development of social networks, participation and involvement in meaningful psychosocial activities, such as education, employment, voluntary work (in their community), cultural and political activities. Whilst some make attempts to integrate with their local community, many find themselves socially isolated. Therefore, an holistic approach, which involves the development and use of a variety of social support networks, should be adopted when working with asylum seekers and refugees.

Farouq's story

Farouq was a 30-year-old male of Iraqi Kurdish origin, referred by his GP. He presented with low mood, suicidal thoughts, low confidence, low self-esteem, sleep difficulties, frequent nightmares and a marked social phobia, as a result of his experiences whilst incarcerated and tortured by the security forces in Iraq under Saddam Hussein's regime. Farouq was a photographer and artist, and became involved in the opposition movement, producing anti-government literature. He was subsequently arrested and detained for over three months, underwent prolonged interrogations, frequent beatings with electric cables, dousing in cold water, sustaining physical trauma of his genitalia as a result of physical abuse. In addition, he was also suspended off the floor for hours from a banister or from his cell windows with his arms bent backwards, a common form of torture used by the Iraqi intelligence services. He was twice taken to hospital when he was no longer able to withstand the torture and collapsed, only to be revived and returned to prison. He was eventually freed after three months and subsequently fled the country to the UK. There was no previous history of psychiatric problems and the anti-depressants from his GP had begun to have a positive effect, albeit small, on his mood. At assessment, his asylum case was ongoing and inevitably this presented him with further very real anxieties and uncertainties about his future.

Farouq received a total of 12-hourly sessions of CBT, over a period of six months. A key focus of early sessions was education regarding the development and maintenance of his mental health problems. This was followed with a combination of graded exposure to feared situations, simple anxiety management techniques, anti-depressant medication and involvement with community resources and activities. The use of EMDR was also used with Farouq, to treat the traumatic memories arising from the torture. Through early discussions, he was able to see the link between his torture experiences, his loss of confidence and self-esteem, which then led to his phobic anxiety in social situations. He was also able to make connections with regards to his symptoms and emotional responses. For example, he was given explanations as to how this pattern developed through avoidance and this was illustrated with simple flow diagrams demonstrating cause and effect, using specific examples from his own experience.

The common reactions to torture, and this presentation in others with similar experiences, were also discussed, thus allowing him to see that his reactions were not 'abnormal'. There was also careful negotiation concerning his goals, especially to determine what would be realistic and achievable. For example, regarding the elimination of symptoms, he was encouraged to accept that in the initial phase of therapy, whilst there would very likely be a reduction in the potency or impact of the symptoms, that the aim of therapy would be to enable him to come to terms with his experience, rather than 'get over it'. He was also encouraged to identify ways in which he would know that things were improving and these became his 'targets', e.g. one of his targets was to be able to 'contribute to meetings and activities at the refugee community centre'. It must be noted that there was a significant improvement in a number of areas of Farouq's functioning, prior to him achieving refugee status.

Another significant issue is the role of memory. A study was undertaken that aimed to investigate the consistency of autobiographical memory of people seeking asylum, to test the assumption that discrepancies in asylum-seeker's accounts of persecution could mean that they are fabricating their stories. The results indicated that for participants with high levels of post-traumatic stress, the number of discrepancies increased with the length of time between interviews. In addition, accounts were more likely to be inconsistent in details that the individual considered as peripheral to their experience, rather than the details they considered to be central to the traumatic event.

For example, dates, times and other details are less likely to be remembered than say the details surrounding their detention, torture, rape, etc. Therefore, inconsistent recall does not necessarily imply the individual is fabricating their accounts of torture or other traumatic experience.

The patient's legal status also makes a difference to treatment outcomes because of the uncertainty surrounding status, and fears of return for those still awaiting asylum decisions. This inevitably impacts on therapeutic progress because the individual is focused on realistic fears for the future and therefore often unable to focus on the 'here and now'. Furthermore, the therapeutic interventions, such a CBT and other approaches, would be inadvisable where the patient is home-less or destitute (which can often be the case, depending on the current asylum laws). In such cases, therapeutic engagement needs to be more focused on creating and fostering a safe environment and the provision of practical support.

Other recent developments in the field have been the development of narrative exposure therapy (NET) (Schauer and colleagues 2005). NET has been developed as an integration of cognitive behavioural therapy (CBT) and testimony therapy (TT), a short-term psychological treatment method that was especially developed for survivors of torture and other severe human rights' violations. TT aims at the construction of a detailed and coherent report of the survivor's biography, including an explicit description of the traumatic events. The written testimony created by the survivor, in co-operation with a therapist, is used for documentary and political purposes in support of the survivor. The procedures of CBT and TT share many common features. As in CBT, prolonged exposure to the traumatic material is realized through reporting about it. This promotes the habituation of emotional and physiological reactions to reminders of the traumatic events and so reduces symptoms. But the focus of TT is not on the patient overcoming fears related to their experiences, but on the reconstruction of the shattered autobiographical memories of the traumatic experiences. NET is therefore a combination of these two approaches and has been used success-fully in many cross-cultural settings, again by working closely with, and train-ing, local professionals, especially teachers. It has been also developed for children and again used in the wake of recent disasters and in refugee camps (see Appendix 3 for website details).

Working with interpreters—some guidelines for mental health workers

- When booking the interpreter, try to provide as much information as possible to help the interpreting service to ensure they send an appropriate interpreter. For example, it is important not just to match the language, but to consider gender and ethnic affiliations. It is important for health workers to have a good working alliance with the interpreter, as well as with the patient.

- Check that the interpreter is acceptable to the patient—an obvious example where this might not be the case would be a male interpreter working with a female patient who has been raped. Also, interpreters sometimes speak the same language, but belong to a hostile ethnic group.

- Since the interpreter may well know a great deal more than the therapist about the patient's culture and background, they can also be an invaluable source of information about how the patient is likely to respond to particular questions or lines of enquiry.

- Patients tend to look at the therapist when he or she is speaking, but look at the interpreter when they themselves are speaking. This reduces the sense of having a direct conversation with the patient, and underlines the fact that the interpreter is a third person in the session, whose sensitivity and responsiveness will have an impact on your work.

- Allow enough time for the interview, as working with an interpreter takes longer, so usually allow 1½–2 hours for a session.

- Before commencing the appointment, it is important that the therapist explains their particular treatment model, how it works and informs the interpreter about the style of interpretation they require to the interpreter.

- Topics covered in the interview are often distressing. Where possible, before the interview, the interpreter should be provided with background information about the patient, including the subject matter likely to be covered. A pre-interview briefing will also give the interpreter the opportunity to brief you on possible cultural issues that might arise in the context of the discussion and any issues they have themselves in relation to the content to be discussed.

- Before the start of the appointment, consider seating arrangements so everyone can be properly and appropriately involved in the interview. This is particularly an issue for family appointments, or appointments where there are likely to be several people in the room.

- If you have any concerns about an interpreter (e.g. the language or cultural match between the interpreter and patient, or you felt that there may be a tension between the interpreter and patient), it is helpful to let the interpreting service know this. This will help the service to find a more appropriate interpreter for the patient in the future, and support the service's quality monitoring.

- Ensure that the interpreter is aware of confidentiality, and has explained to the patient that he/she will treat everything discussed in the interview as strictly confidential.

- During the interview use straightforward language, avoiding complex terminology or jargon.

- Make time available at the end of the session to discuss the case and the interpreter's feelings during the session. This can be brief and will allow the interpreter to give the therapist any additional perspectives he or she may have on the therapeutic encounter. (For example, the interpreter may have noticed that the patient was inhibited from speaking about something, perhaps in line with cultural norms.) The 'de-brief' should also help the interpreter to mentally 'exit' the appointment and relationship with the patient. The interpreter may need support to set boundaries so that they can exit their relationship with the patient at the end of the appointment. (For example, making sure the interpreter does not have to leave the building with the patient.)

Working with asylum seekers and refugees—some guidelines for interpreters

- Therapy sessions are different from psychiatric assessment sessions. An important part of the work with people who have experienced traumatic events often includes the disclosure of shameful feelings and thoughts. This can only be done when trust has been established. This makes it important for them to have the same interpreter, wherever possible, over a course of treatment. It is important to let the therapist know as far in advance as possible about times when you will not be available, such as absences due to other work commitments, holidays and so on.

- As with all health-interpreting appointments, everything discussed in the sessions is confidential. It is important that patients are aware of this and feel confident that you will treat everything as confidential.

- Most therapists prefer interpreters, where possible, to use the 'first person' when translating the patient's words. You may like to check this with the therapist before you start the appointment; sometimes it is acceptable to convey the patient's story in the third person.

- It is important to translate everything the patient says, even if it seems irrelevant to what is being discussed at the time, but share any observations you may have about that experience.

- As an interpreter, you probably know much more than the therapist about the patient's culture and cultural ways of thinking. This knowledge may be very important for the therapist to know. For example, it may help him or her to understand why the patient engages or responds to treatment in a certain way. If you have additional information that you think it would be helpful for the therapist to know, please let them know. However, when doing so, it is important to be clear about when you are interpreting what the patient has said and when you are offering your own opinion.

- As with all interpreting assignments, you should not start discussions with the patient or give direct advice, without first discussing it with the therapist in the first instance. The patient has to make decisions for him or herself.

- Often the phrasing of questions is extremely important, so you should translate as directly as possible without adding, subtracting or putting questions into another form.

- Try not to make open questions into leading questions (i.e. questions that require a yes/no answer). For example, an open question is 'How are you feeling?'; a leading question would be 'Are you feeling OK?'

- Silence during the sessions may be meaningful. Try not to repeat questions or 'push' the patient unless the therapist asks you to do so.

- If the patient asks you not to tell the therapist something, please tell the therapist that they have said this, before the patient has told you what it is they want you not to interpret.

- It can understandable and common for the patient to become upset. The therapist and interpreter should simply acknowledge and validate these feelings. Therefore, when the patient is upset try to resist the urge to comfort the patient directly through touch or by saying, for example, 'it will be OK, don't cry'.

- Therapists are aware that it is not always possible to provide an exact word-for-word translation. Please explain to the therapist why a particular question is hard to ask in a language and suggest possible alternatives that are more appropriate.

- If you have any concerns about the patient, please tell the therapist.

- If you have questions or do not understand what the therapist is doing or why they are asking certain questions, then please ask the therapist at the end of the session when the patient has left. It is important that you have an understanding of what is happening.

- It is important to be aware that the work often involves discussing and describing highly disturbing and distressing situations, and that this may well have an emotional effect on you. Try to find ways of taking care of yourself emotionally when doing this work. In addition to this, the therapist should make time available at the end of the session to discuss the case and your own feelings during the session; this kind of debriefing can help you to manage difficult feelings about the session when you leave. Please ask your therapist to help you if you are experiencing any particular difficulties as a result of the work you have been doing.

Trauma and culture—the work of humanitarian aid agencies

The past decade has seen an increasing focus and consensus on the importance of providing what has become known as 'psychosocial support' following disasters and complex emergencies. Many non-governmental organizations (NGOs) have been actively involved in the delivery of psychosocial support programmes

(PSPs, sometimes also referred to as psychological support programmes) in varied contexts and settings, whether it is following natural disasters, as in the case of the recent Tsunami, or in the wake of armed conflict. The term 'psycho-social' has become the preferred term when describing interventions designed to positively impact on the mental health needs of those individuals and communities affected by complex emergencies and will, therefore, be used throughout this chapter. In addition, the field of psychosocial interventions is relatively young and inevitably there have been calls to determine the evidence base for such interventions. There have also been critiques of the notion of PSP, as there is a view that many communities affected by complex emergencies are resilient and thus have an innate capacity to heal themselves without external intervention. Inevitably, there have also been critiques of the appropriateness and what has often been perceived as the 'medicalized' nature of such interventions.

It is important to understand that individuals, communities and societies, not only cope with, but also have the innate ability to adapt to, adversity and to focus psychosocial interventions at building on these strengths. In 1991 the International Federation of Red Cross and Red Crescent Societies (IFRC) launched the Psychological Support Programme (PSP) as a cross-cutting programme under the Health and Care Division. To assist the IFRC with the implementation of the programme, the Danish Red Cross and IFRC established the Reference Centre for Psychological Support as a centre of excellence in 1993. From November 2004 the centre changed its name to the Reference Centre (RC) for Psychosocial Support, which has the following guiding principles (IFRC Reference Centre for Psychosocial Support 2006):

- ♦ assisting local initiatives, which will lead to a durable and meaningful change in the psychological well-being of people affected by disasters and stressful life events;

- ♦ collaborating with Red Cross/Red Crescent National Societies to build sustainable psychosocial support programmes that are based on genuine local ownership, avoiding the creation of aid -dependent parallel structures;

- ♦ working on the basis of locally identified needs, rather than on the reflexes of the aid community;

- ♦ paying special attention to women and children, who are often the most vulnerable groups in a post-conflict situation, as well as to families with missing members;

- ♦ any discussion on the relationship between humanitarian aid providers and recipients should be based on the concept of respect for the prevailing culture and its mental health or psychosocial healing practices.

Psychosocial interventions and enhancing resilience in complex emergencies

If there is a recognition and acknowledgement that in complex emergencies, such as major disasters, especially those involving severe injuries, bereavement and loss, there will indeed be mental health consequences for many survivors. This would be specially so where the social infrastructure has been compromised, whatever mental health systems existed prior to the emergency that may be insufficient to meet the multifaceted needs of communities affected. Mollica and colleagues (2004), only a few days before the Asian tsunami of 2004, urged countries throughout the world to prepare themselves to deal with 'Mental health in complex emergencies'. It is noteworthy that the authors were not calling for armies of counsellors to be drafted in or for Western models of therapy to be utilized, but acknowledging the impact that disasters can have on individuals, families and communities.

The concept of PSP has become firmly established in the repertoire of humanitarian organizations' interventions following complex emergencies. There is an expectation that individuals and communities following catastrophe are resilient but, there is also an understanding borne out by a considerable body of evidence that there are mental health consequences for some survivors. The loss of life and forced migration suffered by many communities following the Asian tsunami, focused national and international agencies on the need to provide appropriate psychosocial care from the very beginning. The early arguments and criticisms surrounding PSP and early interventions paled into insignificance when faced by the urgent need to reduce distress and prevent the development of longer term mental health problems. In the wake of the death, destruction, multiple bereavements and losses, including homes and livelihoods, doing nothing was not an option. Lessons had also been learned following the mental health response after the earthquake that devastated the city of Barn in Southern Iran, destroying 85% of the city. An estimated 26,000 people were killed and a further 30,000 injured. This response was delivered early and was the product of much planning and preparation for just such a disaster. Knowing that the region was vulnerable to earthquakes, the Department of Mental Health in the Ministry of Health in Iran, in collaboration with the Iranian Red Crescent, started conducting a series of workshops for relief workers in the basic skills of psychosocial support. Further training was also facilitated by UNICEF and the Centre for Crisis Psychology in Norway (Yule 2006).

This example is of course one of among many illustrating that PSPs do not focus on PTSD and are not restricted to a conventional Eurocentric view of suffering and distress. All PSPs are designed in collaboration with local agencies and communities, especially those conducted through the International Red Cross and Red Crescent Societies' Reference Centre for Psychosocial Support. A key element is, and always has been, the facilitation and enhancement of local resources and communities, together with capacity building. Requests for PSPs come from a wide variety of Red Cross and Red Crescent National Societies; a recent example has been within the Somali Red Crescent, which has been developing a culturally sensitive framework for the development and delivery of psychosocial training for its volunteers. In many developing countries the local Red Cross/Red Crescent Society often provides basic health and social care, something in the West that is often taken for granted.

Some have argued that the transfer of Western concepts and techniques, e.g. to war-affected societies, risks perpetuating the colonial status of non-Western mind-sets, as every culture has its own frameworks for mental health and norms for help-seeking at times of crisis. This argument is based on making distinctions between Western 'eurocentric' cultures and cultures in non-industrialized countries, and while it may appear a straightforward distinction, it is far from being the case. Many societies have chosen to adapt mental health concepts developed by Western psychology and prefer corresponding intervention methods, often in combination with traditional healing, as has been seen in South Africa. Similarly, in many rural areas in European countries, traditional healing techniques for physical and mental complaints have remained popular.

There is evidence that there are some instances whereby an integrated model of intervention, using the framework described above, has had significant utility. As referred to earlier, following the earthquake of 2003, in Bam, Iran, the Children and War Recovery Manual (see Appendix 3 for website details) was adapted with local collaboration and used by the psychosocial teams, based on previous experiences and training. This formed the basis for trauma counselling interventions based on cognitive behavioural exercises and included brief group exercises over four sessions with about 960 children and 742 adults. About 1500 local mental health professionals and teachers were trained to provide brief interventions. The evaluations and post-intervention questionnaires and clinician reports indicated that 85% (some 55,000) of the survivors benefited from the sessions (Yule 2006). Many interventions utilize psycho-educational strategies, such as information about the psychological impact of traumatic events and related supportive advice. Support and guidance are likely to cover reassurance about immediate distress, information about the likely course of symptoms, strategies for effective coping, health and psychosocial support in emergency settings. The aim is to systemize the field by development of coherent practice-based guidance. This work is currently being done by the Inter-Agency Standing Committee (IASC) task force on Mental Health and Psychosocial Support in Emergency settings (IASC 2006). The IASC is a unique inter-agency forum for co-ordination, policy development and decision-making involving the key UN and non-UN humanitarian partners. The IASC was established in June 1992 in response to a United Nations General Assembly Resolution on the strengthening of humanitarian assistance. The General Assembly Resolution affirmed its role as the primary mechanism for inter-agency co-ordination of humanitarian assistance. Under the leadership of the IASC, the United Nations develops humanitarian policies, agrees on a clear division of responsibility for the various aspects of humanitarian assistance, identifies and addresses gaps in response, and advocates for effective application of humanitarian principles. Together with the Executive Committee for Humanitarian Affairs (ECHA), the IASC forms the key strategic co-ordination mechanism among major humanitarian agencies.

Psychosocial support following disasters: a case study

On 8 October 2005, a powerful earthquake measuring 7.6 on the Richter scale hit Northern Pakistan and Northern India; the tremors were felt across the region from Kabul in Afghanistan to Delhi. In less than a minute, whole towns and villages were reduced to rubble and landslides had washed away roads and villages on mountain sides. The death toll was more than 80,000, with over 70,000 people injured and 2.6 million people made homeless, with 145,000 being internally displaced in official and *ad hoc* refugee camps. The European Commission Humanitarian Office (ECHO) funded a Psychosocial Programme following the disaster, as the Government of Pakistan, and all relevant stakeholders involved in the relief operation, recognized the urgency of addressing not only the physical and material needs of those affected but also the emotional and psychosocial needs of the population. The funding allowed the Danish Red Cross (DRC) and the Pakistan Red Crescent Society (PRCS), supported by the IFRC to initiate a Psychosocial Programme in four refugee camps in the North-West frontier and in Islamabad in November 2005. The initial assessment, carried out immediately after the earthquake, found the disaster had also caused enormous psychological distress because of significant loss of life, shelter and livelihood, not to mention multiple losses in many cases.

The immediate priority following the earthquake was to provide food, shelter and medical aid to all those affected. The majority of the population in the area affected by the earthquake lived in remote and scattered villages with a limited and basic infrastructure in terms of communication, transport and other services. The small and isolated communities affected, sustained a living through the land, often eking out a basic and simple existence. The literacy rate in the most affected areas was low, with women leading secluded lives, often rarely interacting with the outside world other than their extended family. In addition, some of the affected areas had been isolated as a result of the long-lasting conflict between India and Pakistan in Kashmir. The harsh winter conditions hampered immediate reconstruction, prevented the population from regaining their livelihoods and other day-to-day activities. A large part of the affected population also had to spend the winter months in temporary camps away from their place of origin.

The psychosocial team's assessment indicated that many were experiencing what would be considered normal responses to a disaster of such proportion.

Many felt disbelief at what had happened, finding it difficult to absorb the enormity of the situation and assess the damage and loss for themselves, their families and communities. Initially the emphasis was on practical issues, such as recovering the remains of loved ones, arranging burial ceremonies and other cultural rituals. In this remote area of Pakistan, religion plays an important part in the traditional lifestyle of these isolated communities.

At assessment, the psychosocial team was able to establish many of the challenges presented when organizing a PSP to facilitate culturally appropriate coping strategies. It was decided at an early stage that it was of great importance to involve individuals, families and communities within the camp in the decisions regarding psychosocial initiatives, so that they could express what they regarded as helpful in the facilitation of a healing process and to enhance their natural resilience. The team were also very aware of the significance of religion and the role of women in a very traditional and rural setting of Pakistan.

The programme began in November 2005 and was implemented within the biggest refugee camps, utilizing 16 PRCS field workers, a programme manager and a field team co-ordinator. All these individuals were recruited and trained using context-specific psychosocial models and working in collaboration with local NGOs who agreed to provide training, professional supervision and support to field workers during the project period. Within three months, four teams had generated awareness about the psychological reactions to trauma, established a variety of social activities and organized volunteers in four of the large camps. The volunteers were initially supported until they felt able to work independently, before other similar activities were established in surrounding villages and communities. Activities were all based on participatory assessments and knowledge gained from focused interviews and multiple meetings with the target communities. The most common activity was psycho-educational sessions for different groups, e.g. children of different ages, women and men. Social activities were also initiated, aimed at creating a safe and culturally appropriate environment, where different groups could meet, share problems, concerns and be actively involved in the recovery and rehabilitation process.

The PRCS had not previously been involved in psychosocial activities and subsequently did not have any staff who were trained in this area, or who could be transferred to the new programme. In the event, all field workers were new employees having been newly introduced to the PRCS and the Red Crescent movement, receiving intensive training in required knowledge and skills. The psychosocial team found that experience and lessons learned from other PSPs meant it was important to create specific modules designed for each of the project areas. For example, women in the affected areas, not being used to attending groups where they shared feelings and feedback, were in groups facilitated by women. Widows and orphans were often absorbed into extended families and not seen as particularly vulnerable. However, the new dynamic created by social, emotional and economic situations in a new family can be extremely problematic and result in violence and abuse. Therefore, this was a significant challenge and was addressed by using field workers and volunteers drawn from the local communities. At the time of writing, the projects continue and there are plans to further develop expertise for staff, to strengthen the PRCS and engage in capacity building, ultimately incorporating psychosocial support and activities within the PRCS heath department.

Conclusion

As can be seen the concept of trauma across cultures is a complex subject for a variety of reasons, but there is an acknowledgement of the human condition. The impact of traumatic events on individuals, families and communities seems well understood by people from non-Western cultural backgrounds, even in the face of variations in concepts of health and healing. There is reason to believe that reactions to traumatic events do have a degree of universality. The International Federation of Red Cross and Red Crescent Society's Reference Centre for Psycho-social Support has been responding to requests from different countries to establish psychosocial programmes to complement other activities, such as community-based first-aid. Across cultures, human beings have similar reactions to distressing, stressful and traumatic events—to those reactions but *their responses may differ—as may interventions.*

8

Growth following adversity

> ## ➲ Key points
>
> ◆ People often report perceiving benefits following trauma.
>
> ◆ Frequently, people mention improved relationships, changes in life philosophy and shifts in how they think about themselves.
>
> ◆ Perceived benefits arise from the struggle to make sense of what has happened.
>
> ◆ Perceiving benefits can help people cope and can lead to improved outcomes.
>
> ◆ Therapists can help people to explore what benefits they can find following trauma.

Introduction

Throughout human history, a number of literatures, religions and philosophies have conveyed the idea that there are benefits to be found following exposure to adversity, extreme stress and trauma. However, it is only relatively recently that these benefits have become a focus for research. Initially there was some debate and controversy over the idea of positive growth following trauma. But there is now convincing evidence that people often experience benefits following stress and trauma.

These benefits have been described in a number of different ways; for example, labelled as adversarial growth, benefit-finding, flourishing, heightened existential awareness, perceived benefits, positive by-products, positive changes, positive meaning, post-traumatic growth, self-renewal, stress-related growth, thriving and transformational coping. These terms have been used interchangeably to refer, not just to recovery following stressful and traumatic events, but how events can sometimes serve as the springboard to a higher level of psychological well-being.

The idea of benefits is different to the idea of resilience. Like trees caught in a massive wind, which immediately spring back to their original shape when the wind dies down, resilient people are unaffected by trauma. In contrast, growth-ful people are affected by the trauma, and change as a result. Three broad but related dimensions of benefit finding have been discussed. First, relationships are enhanced in some way; for example, that people now value their friends and family more, and feel an increased compassion and kindness toward others. Secondly, people change their views of themselves in some way; for example, that they have a greater sense of personal resiliency, wisdom and strength, per-haps coupled with a greater acceptance of their vulnerabilities and limitations. Third, there are reports of changes in life philosophy; for example, finding a fresh appreciation for each new day, shifts in understanding of what really mat-ters in life, Sometimes, there may be changes in spiritual beliefs. For example, for Karen, a survivor of childhood abuse, it was the recognition that change is inevitable, being able to accept the past and to be able to live in the present:

> It has been a time of great contrasts—anguish and despair followed by real joy and confidence. I feel as if I have crossed a bridge and now on the other side, but still finding my feet... I know though that life is change and one of the ways I have changed is a much greater sense of living in the present, being present now and accepting that everything changes and ultimately dies....

Living in the present was also mentioned by Isobella, another survivor, who described how she now views life as a positive learning process, and to be her-self. However, she also adds that her biggest change is in her attitude to death:

> I enjoy everyday to the full, I don't worry about silly things anymore and if something is important to me I make an effort to do or say something about it. I speak my mind and have no regrets about anything... I realize now that, however unjust or unfair, Robert's death was that this is part of life. Sometimes things that seem unfair have to happen and, although I'd rather he was alive, I have learnt a great deal from the experience.... The biggest thing I've gained from this is that I don't fear death....

Measuring positive change following trauma

Various psychological self-report tests have been developed to assess positive changes and personal growth following adversity One of these is the Changes in Outlook Positive (CiOP) Questionnaire (Figure 8.1). The CiOP is designed to assess positive views of the world in the aftermath of adversity. Each of the statements in the questionnaire was made by people who experienced extremely stressful and traumatic events in their lives.

The amount of benefit that people experience varies between different research studies, depending on the types of groups studied, the context and experiences of those in the studies and the type of research methods used. However, it would be expected that anywhere between 30 and 70% of people may typically experi-ence some form of benefit following traumatic events. In one study it was found

Consider possible positive changes in your outlook that may have come about following a recent or past traumatic experience. Please read each statement and indicate, by circling the number in the appropriate box, how much you agree or disagree with it AT THE PRESENT TIME:

1 = Strongly disagree, 2 = Disagree, 3 = Disagree a little, 4 = Agree a little, 5 = Agree, 6 = Strongly agree.

	Strongly disagree	Disagree	Disagree a little	Agree a little	Agree	Strongly agree
1. I don't take life for granted anymore.	1	2	3	4	5	6
2. I value my relationships much more now.	1	2	3	4	5	6
3. I feel more experienced about life now.	1	2	3	4	5	6
4. I don't worry about death at all anymore.	1	2	3	4	5	6
5. I live everyday to the full now.	1	2	3	4	5	6
6. I look upon each day as a bonus.	1	2	3	4	5	6
7. I'm a more understanding and tolerant person now.	1	2	3	4	5	6
8. I have a greater faith in human nature now.	1	2	3	4	5	6
9. I no longer take people or things for granted.	1	2	3	4	5	6
10. I value other people more now.	1	2	3	4	5	6
11. I am more determined to succeed in life now.	1	2	3	4	5	6

To calculate your score, add up your responses to all eleven items.

The lowest possible score is 11 and the highest possible score is 66.

Scores of 44 or over can be taken to indicate some amount of positive change.

Figure 8.1 Changes in Outlook Positive (CiOP) Questionnaire. Joseph, S., Williams, R., & Yule, W. (1993). *Journal of Traumatic Stress*, **6**, 271–279. Reprinted with permission of John Wiley & Sons, Inc. See Appendix 1 for full version.

that 58% of people in a national American survey reported benefits two months after the terrorist attacks in New York on 11 September 2001.

Positive changes are not usually reported in the very immediate aftermath but at some time later. In the immediate aftermath, people are confused and disorientated, and may be experiencing shock. In the subsequent weeks they may be emotionally confused and experiencing post-traumatic stress. Until the person has reached a certain emotional equilibrium, it is likely to be too soon to think about benefits. We would always be careful about even introducing the topic of benefits to clients. What we find is that when the time is right for the person, they are likely to introduce the topic themselves, if we give them the space to do so.

Benefits are likely to be present alongside psychological distress. It is not that the experience of benefits is mutually exclusive to other more negative psychological consequences. It seems that to some extent distress helps to trigger the search for benefits, but as people find benefits, this in turn helps them to cope with the distress (see Anna's story).

Anna's story

Anna is a 26-year-old woman who was the victim of a violent rape by four men, whilst on holiday on a Greek island. Stuart, her boyfriend, who was with her at the time, was also badly physically assaulted in the attack. The couple did report the assault, which was a high-profile case, making the national and international news. On return to the UK, Anna reported it to the British police and was subsequently seen by a forensic surgeon and went through the normal process that many rape survivors have to undergo in the UK. She was persuaded to return to Greece to try and take the matter further, which she subsequently did but no-one was arrested or charged with the assault. As can be expected, the return to the place of the assault was a significant re-traumatizing factor for her.

In the months and years that followed Anna developed significant symptoms of post-traumatic stress disorder and a prolonged period of depression. She had put on a significant amount of weight, increased her alcohol consumption, had given up her job, developed a range of avoidance behaviour, could not stay alone in the house and had started sleeping with a carving knife under her pillow. By this time she had married Stuart, who had been supportive throughout. Their feelings for each other had not changed as a result of their experience, if anything they had grown closer together. They eventually had a child and the subsequent birth of her daughter, Claire, prompted Anna to see her GP, as she felt that she would not be able to look after her daughter, given the problems she was having, and this prompted her to seek treatment. A referral was subsequently made and Anna received 12 sessions of trauma-focused cognitive behavioural therapy (CBT),

> which included EMDR. She made significant progress and when seen at a one-year follow-up appointment she reported that she had made 90% improvement overall, was working, going out with friends on a regular basis, could stay alone at home when Stuart was working away and had discontinued her anti-depressants.

Whilst Anna's story is shocking and would affect anyone in similar circumstances, she worked hard to bring about change in her life, in order to improve the quality of her own life and that of her daughter and family. She realized she could not continue with her life the way she had been doing. There is, however, a further tragic postscript to her story, which could be seen as illustrative of post-traumatic growth. Four years to the day following the assault, whilst on holiday with her family, Stuart literally dropped dead at the dining table at the holiday cottage on the second day of their holiday. Whilst Anna quite naturally experienced a traumatic bereavement, over the years she has come through this, come to terms with Stuart's loss and has met and re-married. Whilst this brief vignette does not do full justice to her story or her resourcefulness in the face of overwhelming adversity, the following quotes below taken from an interview some years following Stuart's loss are illuminating and could be seen as illustrative of post-traumatic growth.

....what happened in Greece was such a huge trauma... a huge thing—but I came through that and I thought after Greece I would never be able to live a normal life again ever. Then I was proved wrong because obviously with the stuff we did together I got my life back to normality and then, with Stuart dying, it gave me belief in myself that I could come through that, and it has also made me think that life's very short and we have got to make the most of what you've got....

I think over the last year, obviously there have been changes and my whole outlook on life is different because I had always thought I would have a big family, and I know that has changed now, but I can accept that that is the way it is now. I think I don't look as far into the future now, I just take.... Not every day as it comes, but just take short periods of time to see what happens, rather than planning the future. I think that has changed me as a person.

Sometimes I think—I really can't believe that I am in this point in my life, laughing and happy—and even when I got out of the car today and walked up to see you—it is a long way from the time when I first came to see you and can't believe I come on my own and I wondered myself how I cope. I came because I have to, because I feel I have no choice, because I have got Claire who has to be able to live her life happily, and I also feel now—and I didn't always feel like this—that life is for living and I have got no choice. I am here, so I can either enjoy it and get on with it or be miserable.

Findings from the research on growth following adversity

Studies have reported benefits following a range of stressful and traumatic events; for example, bereavement, accidents and disasters, chronic and life-threatening illness, sexual, physical and emotional abuse in childhood, sexual assault, and war and conflict. Research has also begun to document why some people and not others are more likely to report benefits. Are some people more inclined to find benefits in their experience? The answer seems to be 'yes'. Studies of groups of people following adversity suggested that, while growth is not always reported, at least some people reported growth in *all of the studies*, suggesting that all life events have the potential to be triggers for positive change.

◆ Positive changes were more likely in women compared to men.

◆ Younger people were more likely than older people to report positive changes.

◆ People who were better educated were more likely to report positive changes.

◆ People with higher incomes were more likely to report positive change.

◆ Personality seemed to be important too. People who were more extraverted, open to experience, agreeable, conscientious and emotionally stable, were more likely to report positive changes.

◆ More optimistic people were more likely to report positive changes.

◆ People who are more able to actively cope with problems in their life are more likely to experience positive changes.

◆ People who were more able to deal with their emotions, such as by seeking out support from others, were more likely to report positive changes.

◆ People who are able to use positive reinterpretation as a way of coping were more likely to report positive changes.

◆ People who use more acceptance coping strategies were more likely to report positive changes.

◆ People who have more positive emotions were more likely to report positive changes.

◆ People who are more intrinsically religious were more likely to report positive change.

◆ People most likely to experience growth have more nurturing, accepting, validating, loving, social relationships. These people, it seems, have a natural tendency to make positive changes in their lives.

But although some people seem to be more likely to find benefits, this does not mean that other people will not be able to. We can learn from those who do find benefits about what they do and use this knowledge to help others.

The importance of this avenue of investigation is seen in the groundbreaking work of Glenn Affleck and colleagues who found that perceived benefits at seven weeks following a heart attack significantly predicted less chance of a heart attack recurrence and lower general health problems eight years later, when patients were followed-up. Other studies since have also shown that those who perceive benefits are less likely to have problems of depression, anxiety and post-traumatic stress subsequently.

Tedeschi and Calhoun, two of the pioneers of this area of research, suggest that traumatic events serve as significant challenges by shattering prior goals, beliefs, leading to self reflection, as people try to make sense of what has happened. Although this can be distressing, this self-reflection process is indicative of mental activity that is directed at rebuilding the individual's beliefs, ideas and values. This reflective process is influenced by social support networks that provide sources of comfort and relief, as well as being influenced by new coping behaviours and available options for the construction of new ideas and beliefs after the trauma. As successful coping aids adaptation, the initial self-reflection that was characterized by its automatic nature, shifts towards a more constructive mental activity characterized by the development of a narrative, part of which may be the search for meaning, eventually leading to growth.

Seen from this perspective, growth, rather than an illness or disorder, can be the outcome of the traumatic stress response.

Considerations for therapy

In our own work we have emphasized that growth following adversity is a normal and natural process, one that people are innately motivated toward. The task of the therapist is not to supply people with the answers to their questions and tell them what meaning to find in their experience. People will do this for themselves. The task is to provide the safe supportive opportunity for this to take place.

Experimental studies to test whether the principles of growth might somehow be introduced as part of a clinical intervention are encouraging. For example, a study that randomly assigned breast cancer patients to one of two groups, either to write about the facts of the cancer experience or to write about their positive thoughts and feelings regarding the experience, found that those assigned to write about positive experiences had significantly fewer medical appointments for cancer-related problems three months later.

Therapists should be aware of the potential for positive change in their clients following stress and trauma. But it must also be recognized that adversity does not lead to positive change for everyone. Therefore, therapists need to be careful not to inadvertently imply that the person has in some way failed by not making more of their experience, or that there is anything inherently positive in the person's experience. Personal growth after trauma should be viewed as originating not from the event, but from within the person themselves through the process of their struggle with the event and its aftermath. In order to further investigate and aid clinical work into this important topic, we have developed a new tool, the Psychological Well-Being – Post-traumatic Changes Questionnaire (PWB-PTCQ: see appendix 2). The PWB-PTCQ is an 18 item questionnaire that is designed to assess change on six domains: self-acceptance, autonomy, purpose in life, relationships, sense of mastery, and personal growth.

Conclusion

For those dealing with trauma and losses, understanding that what they are going through has the potential to be a springboard for something positive can be a hopeful message. It can also seem unrealistic and naïve to those in the midst of suffering. This is understandable but it is our experience with hundreds of clients who have sought help that although the journey can be long and arduous, it is one that it can be lead to growth.

One of the most remarkable advances in our knowledge of trauma in recent years is that, in the aftermath of the struggle with adversity, it is common to find benefits. The perception of benefits, in turn, may lead to higher levels of psychological functioning and improved health. This is not to overlook the personal devastation of psychological trauma, but equally we must not overlook the fact that psychological trauma does not necessarily lead to a damaged life. Simply being aware of the possibility of benefits can offer hope to people.

Appendix 1

Negative Changes in Outlook (CiON)

	Strongly Disagee	Disagree	Disagree a little	Agree a little	Agree	Strongly Agree
1. I don't look forward to the future anymore.	1	2	3	4	5	6
2. My life has no meaning anymore.	1	2	3	4	5	6
3. I no longer feel able to cope with things.	1	2	3	4	5	6
4. I fear death very much now.	1	2	3	4	5	6
5. I feel as if something bad is just waiting around the corner to happen.	1	2	3	4	5	6
6. I desperately wish I could turn the clock back to before it happened.	1	2	3	4	5	6
7. I sometimes think it's not worth being a good person.	1	2	3	4	5	6
8. I have very little trust in other people now.	1	2	3	4	5	6
9. I feel very much as if I'm in limbo.	1	2	3	4	5	6
10. I have very little trust in myself now.	1	2	3	4	5	6
11. I feel harder towards other people.	1	2	3	4	5	6

(continued)

	Strongly Disagee	Disagree	Disagree a little	Agree a little	Agree	Strongly Agree
12. I am less tolerant of others now.	1	2	3	4	5	6
13. I am much less able to communicate with other people.	1	2	3	4	5	6
14. Nothing makes me happy anymore.	1	2	3	4	5	6
15. I feel as if I'm dead from the neck downwards.	1	2	3	4	5	6

Strongly disagree = 1, Disagree = 2, Disagree a little = 3, Agree a little = 4, Agree = 5, Strongly Agree = 6.

To calculate the negative change score, add up all your responses to the 15 items above. The lowest you can score is 15, the highest is 90. A number of studies have shown that average scores of people who have experienced trauma are between 27 and 33. The higher your score the more likely it is that you will also experience other problems of posttraumatic stress and impaired general health. Joseph, S., Williams, R., and Yule, W. (1993). *Journal of Traumatic Stress*, **6**, 271–279. Reprinted with permission of John Wiley & Sons, Inc.

Appendix 2

Psychological Well-Being - Post-Traumatic Change Questionnaire (PWB-PTCQ) © Stephen Joseph and Steve Regel (2009)

Think about how you feel about yourself at the present time. Please read each of the following statements and rate how you have changed as a result of the trauma.

5 = Much more so now

4 = A bit more so now

3 = I feel the same about this as before

2 = A bit less so now

1 = Much less so now

_____1. I like myself.

_____2. I have confidence in my opinions.

_____3. I have a sense of purpose in life.

_____4. I have strong and close relationships in my life.

_____5. I feel I am in control of my life.

_____6. I am open to new experiences that challenge me.

_____7. I accept who I am, with both my strengths and limitations.

_____8. I don't worry what other people think of me.

_____9. My life has meaning.

_____10. I am a compassionate and giving person.

_____11. I handle my responsibilities in life well.

_____12. I am always seeking to learn about myself.

_____13. I respect myself.

_____14. I know what is important to me and will stand my ground, even if others disagree.

_____15. I feel that my life is worthwhile and that I play a valuable role in things.

_____16. I am grateful to have people in my life who care for me.

_____17. I am able to cope with what life throws at me.

_____18. I am hopeful about my future and look forward to new possibilities.

Add up your scores to all 18 statements. Scores over 54 indicate the presence of positive change. The maximum score is 90. The higher your score, the more positive change you have experienced.

You may have changed more on some areas than others. Self-acceptance (statements 1, 7, & 13), autonomy (statements 2, 8, & 14), purpose in life (statements 3, 9, & 15), relationships (statements 4, 10, & 16), sense of mastery (statements 5, 11, & 17), and personal growth (statements 6, 12, & 18).

Appendix 3

Useful websites

Aberdeen Centre for Trauma Research, Robert Gordon University, Aberdeen
http://www.rgu.ac.uk/actr/general/page.cfm

American Journal of Psychiatry
http://ajp.psychiatryonline.org/

American Psychological Association
http://www.apa.org

Amnesty International
http://www.amnesty.org.uk/

Anxiety UK
Anxiety UK is the leading UK charity specialising in supporting and helping people affected by a range of anxiety disorders, including PTSD. We aim to provide information, support and understanding via an extensive range of services, and also campaign to raise awareness of anxiety and anxiety disorders nationally.
http://www.anxietyuk.org.uk/

Australasian Society for Traumatic Stress Studies
http://www.astss.org.au/

Australian Centre for Posttraumatic Mental Health
http://www.acpmh.unimelb.edu.ac

Australian Psychological Society
http://www.psychsociety.com.au

BRAKE
http://www.brake.org.uk/

British Association for Behavioural and Cognitive Psychotherapies
http://www.babcp.com/

British Journal of Psychiatry
http://bjp.rcpsych.org/

British Psychological Society
http://www.bps.org.uk/

British Red Cross
http://www.redcross.org.uk/

Canadian Psychiatric Association
http://cpa_apc.org

Canadian Psychological Association
http://www.cpa.org

Centre for Crisis Psychology, Bergen, Norway
http://www.krisepsyk.no/

Centre for Trauma Resilience and Growth, Nottingham
http://www.nottinghamshirehealthcare.nhs.uk/trauma

Children and War
http://www.childrenandwar.org/

Combat Stress
http://www.combatstress.org.uk/

Cruse Bereavement Care
http://www.crusebereavementcare.org.uk/

David Baldwin's Trauma Pages (an excellent portal for trauma related information and resources)
http://www.trauma-pages.com/

Department of Health – Improving Access to Psychological Therapies
http://www.dh.gov.uk/en/Publicationsandstatistics/Publications/
PublicationsPolicyAndGuidance/DH_083150

Disaster Action
http://www.disasteraction.org.uk/

Forced Migration Online
http://www.forcedmigration.org

Harvard Program in Refugee Trauma
http://www.hprt-cambridge.org

Health for Asylum Seekers and Refugees (HARP)
http://www.harpweb.org.uk/

Hostage UK

Hostage UK supports British hostages and their families during and after an overseas kidnapping. We also work with various related organizations to improve their family response and conduct research to enhance public understanding.

www.hostageuk.org

E: administrator@hostageuk.org

Human Rights Watch

http://www.hrw.org

International Comittee of the Red Cross

International Comittee of the Red Cross is an independent, neutral organization ensuring humanitarian protection and assistance for victims of war and other situations of violence.

International Crisis Incident Stress Foundation

http://www.icisf.org

International Federation of Red Cross & Red Crescent Societies

http://www.ifrc.org/

International Federation of Red Cross & Red Crescent Societies
Reference Centre for Psychosocial Support

http://psp.drk.dk/sw2955.asp

International Rehabilitation Centre for Torture Victims

http://www.irct.org

International Society for Traumatic Stress Studies

http://www.istss.org

Medecins Sans Frontieres

http://www.msf.org/

Medical Foundation for the Care of Victims of Torture

http://www.torturecare.org.uk

National Centre for PTSD Washington (and for PILOTS database)

http://www.ncptsd.org/

National Institute for Clinical Excellence (NICE)

http://www.nice.org.uk/

NICE Guidelines PTSD link

http://guidance.nice.org.uk/CG26

Redress

http://www.redress.org/

Refugee Studies Centre, University of Oxford
http://www.rsc.ox.ac.uk

South African Institute for Traumatic Stress
http://www.saits.org.za/

The European Society for Traumatic Stress
http://www.estss.org/

The Inter-Agency Standing Committee (IASC) (The primary mechanism for inter-agency coordination of humanitarian assistance involving the key UN and non-UN humanitarian partners)
http://humanitarianonfo/org/iasc

UK Psychological Trauma Society (UKPTS)
http://www.ukpts.co.uk

UK Resilience
http://www.cabinetoffice.gov.uk/ukresilience.aspx

UK Trauma Group (resources in UK for accessing treatment in local areas)
http://www.uktrauma.org.uk/

United Nations High Commissioner for Refugees (UNHCR)
http://www.unhcr.org

Victim Support
http://www.victimsupport.org.uk

Victim support
www.victimsupport.org.uk
E: chris.wade@victimsupport.org.uk

VIVO Foundation (For Narrative Exposure Therapy - NET)
http://www.vivo.org/

Useful Contact
Dr Anne Eyre
Trauma Training
PO Box 4495
Coventry
CV39BQ
E: anne.eyre@traumatraining.com

Appendix 4

References

American Psychiatric Association (1994) *Diagnostic and Statistical Manual of Mental Disorders* (4th edn). American Psychiatric Press, Washington DC.

Blake D.D., Weathers F.W., Nagy L.M., Kaloupek D.G., Gusman F. D., Charney D.S., Keane, T.M. (1995). The development of a clinician-administered PTSD scale. *Journal of Traumatic Stress* **8**, 75–90.

Brewin C.R., Dalgleish T., Joseph S. (1996) A dual representation theory of posttraumatic stress disorder. *Psychological Review* **103** (4), 670–686.

Brewin C.R. et al (2002) Brief screening instrument for post-traumatic stress disorder. *British Journal of Psychiatry Vol. 181,* 158–162.

Bulman R.J., (1992) *Shattered Assumptions—Towards a New Psychology of Trauma.* Free Press, New York.

Calhoun L.G., Tedeschi R.G. (1999) *Facilitating Post Traumatic Growth: A Clinician's Guide.* Lawrence Erlbaum Associates, London.

Dyregrov A. (1989) Caring for helpers in disaster situations: psychological debriefing. *Disaster Management* **2** (1), 25–30.

Epstein S. (1991) The self concept, the traumatic neurosis, and the structure of the personality. In: Ozer D.J., Healy J.M., Stewart A.J. (eds) *Perspectives in Personality: Vol.13, Part A: Self and Emotion; Part B: Approaches to Understanding Lives.* Jessica Kingsley, Philadelphia, pp.63–98.

Ehlers A., Clark D.M., (2000) A cognitive model of posttraumatic stress disorder. *Behavioural Research and Therapy* **38**, 319–336.

Foa E.B. (1996) *Posttraumatic Stress Diagnostic Scale (PDS).* National Computer Systems, Minneapolis, MN.

Foa E.B., Ehlers A., Clark D.M., Tolin D.F., Orsillo S.M. (1999) The Posttraumatic Cognitions Inventory (PTCI): Development and Validation. *Psychological Assessment* **11** (3), 303–314.

Goldberg, D (1981) *The General Health Questionnaire (GHQ-28).* NFER-Nelson.

Horowitz M., Wilner N., Alvarez W. (1979) Impact of event scale: a measure of subjective stress. *Psychosomatic Medicine* **41** (3), 209–218.

IASC Task Force on Mental Health and Psychosocial Support in Emergency Settings (2006) http://www.humanitarianinfo.org/iasc/content/documents/

Janet P. (1909) *Les Névroses.* Flammarion, Paris.

Joseph, S., Andrews, B., Williams, R., & Yule, W. (1992). Crisis support and psychiatric symptomatology in survivors of the Jupiter cruise ship disaster. *British Journal of Clinical Psychology,* 31, 63–73.

Joseph, S., Williams, R., & Yule, W. (1993). Changes in outlook following disaster: The preliminary development of a measure to assess positive and negative responses. *Journal of Traumatic Stress,* 6, 271–279, with permission.

Mollica R.R., Lopez Cardoza B., Osofsky H.J., Raphael B., Ager A., Salama P. (2004) Mental health in complex emergencies. *Lancet* **364**, 2058–2067.

National Institute for Clinical Excellence (2005) *Post-traumatic Stress Disorder (PTSD): The Management of PTSD in Adults and Children in Primary and Secondary Care.* Gaskell, London (www.nice.org.uk).

Rachman, S., (1980) Emotional processing. *Behaviour Research and Therapy* **18** (1), 51–60.

Reference Centre for Psychosocial Support (2006) Guiding Principles: (http://psp.drk.dk/sw26837.asp)

Stroebe M.S. (1992) Coping with bereavement: a review of the grief work hypothesis. *Omega: Journal of Death and Dying* **26**, 19–42.

Schauer M., Neuner F., Elber T. (2005) *Narrative Exposure Therapy: A Short-Term Intervention for Traumatic Stress Disorders after War, Terror, or Torture*, Vol. 1. Hogrefe and Huber, Massachusetts, pp.1–68.

Yule, W (2006) Theory, training and timing: Psychosocial interventions in complex emergencies. *International Review of Psychiatry* **18** (3), 259–264.

Some useful reading

General

Brewin C.R. (2003) *Post-traumatic Stress Disorder: Malady or Myth?* Yale University Press, New Haven & London.

A very readable overview of the nature of trauma and some of the critiques surrounding PTSD.

Calhoun L.G., Tedeschi R.G. (1999) *Facilitating Post Traumatic Growth: A Clinician's Guide.* Lawrence Erlbaum Associates, London.

Informative and introduces the field of post-traumatic growth, especially useful to counsellors and psychotherapists and useful to general readership because of many examples used

Joseph S., William R., Yule W. (1997) *Understanding Post-traumatic Stress—A Psychosocial Perspective on PTSD and Treatment.* Wiley, Chichester.

A good introductory textbook to the field.

Joseph S., Linley P.A. (eds) (2007) *Trauma, Recovery, and Growth: Positive Psychological Perspectives On Post-Traumatic Stress.* Wiley, Hoeboken.

Especially useful to professionals who want to know more about the latest research and findings in the field of post-traumatic growth.

Herman., JL. (1992) *Trauma and Recovery—From Domestic Abuse to Physical Terror.* Harper Collins, London.

Seen by many as a seminal work. For general readership (as well as professional), a historical and political overview of trauma and explorations of gender and trauma.

van der Kolk B.A., McFarlane A.C., Weisaeth L. (eds) (1996) *Traumatic Stress.* Guilford, New York.

Thorough and comprehensive textbook on all aspects of trauma and PTSD with contributions from leading researchers in the field.

Psycho-social management of disasters

Gibson M. (2006) *Order From Chaos: Responding to Traumatic Event*s (3rd edn). Policy Press, Birmingham.

Very readable and practical text about the impact and management of disasters, especially for those responding in the emergency phases.

International Federation of Red Cross and Red Crescent Societies (published annually) World Disasters Report. Oxford University Press, Oxford.

Good overview of disasters and the international responses, usually with different themes. Useful for statistics and published every year.

Ursano R.J., McCaughy B., Fullerton C. (eds) (1994) *Individual and Community Responses to Disaster.* Cambridge University Press, Cambridge.

Comprehensive textbook on disasters and their aftermath.

Working with refugees

Schauer M., Neuner F., Elbert T. (2005) *Narrative Exposure Therapy: A Short-Term Intervention for Traumatic Stress Disorders after War, Terror or Torture.* Hogrefe & Huber, Washington.

Excellent overview of the theory and application Narrative Exposure Therapy (NET).

Van der Veer G. (1992) *Counselling and Therapy with Refugees - Psychological Problems of Victims of War, Torture and Repression.* Wiley, New York.

Useful and practical text on counselling with refugee populations.

Wilson J.P., Drozdek B. (eds) (2004) *Broken Spirits: The Treatment of Traumatized Asylum Seekers, Refugees, War and Torture Victims.* Brunner-Routledge, New York.

Comprehensive textbook on approaches to working with the populations referred to in the title.

Treatment

Follette V., Ruzek J., Abueg F. (eds) (1998) *Cognitive-Behavioural Therapies for Trauma.* Guilford Press, London.

Some useful chapters, especially an excellent chapter on working with trauma related guilt.

Jehu D. (1988) *Beyond Sexual Abuse—Cognitive Therapy with Women who were Childhood Victims.* Wiley, New York.

Not new, but a good text on understanding how cognitive therapy can be effective with survivors of sexual abuse, with many clinical examples.

Yule W. (ed.) (2003) *Post-Traumatic Stress Disorders: Concepts & Therapy* (3rd edn). Wiley, Chichester.

Excellent overview of concepts such as social support and attribution and their role in the spectrum of trauma responses.

Scott M., Stradling S. (2000) *Counselling for Post-traumatic Stress Disorder* (2nd edn). Sage, London.

A practical guide for the counsellor in general practice or other settings.

Shapiro F., Forrest M.S. (1997) EMDR: *The Breakthrough Therapy For Overcoming Anxiety, Stress and Trauma*. Basic Books, New York.

General introduction on EMDR, suitable for the professional and more informed lay reader.

Trauma and children

Dyregrov A. (1991) *Grief in Children: A Handbook for Adults*. Jessica Kingsley, London.

Excellent for understanding children's responses to grief, very readable and practical.

Harris-Hendriks J., Black D, Kaplan T. (2000) *When Father Kills Mother—Guiding Children Through Trauma and Grief* (2nd edn). Routledge, London.

Very good guide for those working with children and families affected by sudden traumatic bereavement following homicide.

Yule W., Gold A. (1993) *Wise Before the Event : Coping with Crises in Schools*. Calouste Gulbenkian Foundation, London.

For teachers and others—an excellent guide to preparing for and coping with crises in educational settings.

Early interventions for trauma

Dyregov A. (2003) *Psychological Debriefing: A Leader's Guide for Small Group Crisis Intervention*. Chevron Publishing Corporation, Ellicott City.

The best practical guide to the subject of group crisis intervention and debriefing.

Everley G.S, Mitchell J.T. (2008) *Integrative Crisis Intervention and Disaster Mental Health*. Chevron Publishing, Ellicott City, MD.

A general overview of Critical Incident Stress Management and Critical Incident Stress Debriefing- useful for the emergency services.

Raphael B., Wilson J.P. (eds) (2000) *Psychological Debriefing: Theory, Practice and Evidence*. Cambridge University Press.

Academic textbook devoted to the research and practice in the area, with chapters by detractors and supporters of CISM and PD.

The British Psychological Society (BPDS) (2002) *Psychological Debriefing: Professional Practice Board Working Party*. BPS, Leicester.

The BPS's report on Psychological Debriefing which can be found on line at the BPS website Culture/Societies in conflict.

Marsella A.J., Freidman M.J., Gerrity E.T., Scurfield R. (1996) (eds) *Ethnocultural Aspects of Post-traumatic Stress Disorde—Issues, Research and Clinical Applications*. American Psychiatric Press, Washington DC.

A very comprehensive textbook on trauma in different cultural contexts.

Smyth M., Fay M-T. (2000) *Personal Accounts from Northern Ireland's Troubles*. Pluto, London.

Personal stories and testimonies from those affected by the Troubles.

Truth and Reconciliation Commission (TRC) of South Africa Report, Vols. 1–5 (1999) (2nd edn). MacMillan, London.

Comprehensive and moving testimonies and accounts from the TRC proceedings. A fascinating insight into a country trying to come to terms with its past.

Bereavement and grief

Dyregrov K., Dyregrov A. (2008) *Effective Grief and Bereavement Support*. Jessica Kingsley, London.

Does exactly what it says in the title. Up to date and very practical, with lots of suggestions for intervening in different contexts and settings.

Trauma and the law

Napier M., Wheat K. (2002) *Recovering Damages for Psychiatric Injury* (2nd edn). Oxford University Press, Oxford.

Comprehensive overview and guide to the law in relation to psychiatric injury and employer's liability, duty of care etc. Essential reading for solicitors and those preparing psychiatric reports.

Self-help guides

These are books that may be helpful where other problems are present in addition to PTSD or related to the development and maintenance of the problem e.g. obsessive compulsive disorder. They are accessible and practical and can be used as an adjunct to therapy by the therapist and patient.

Kennerley H. (2000) *Overcoming Childhood Trauma: A Self-Help Guide Using Cognitive Behavioural Techniques*. Robinson,London.

Fennell M. (1999) *Overcoming Low Self-Esteem: A Self-Help Guide Using Cognitive Behavioural Techniques*. Robinson, London

Gilbert P. (2000) *Overcoming Depression: A Self-Help Guide Using Cognitive Behavioural Techniques* (2nd edn). Robinson, London.

Silove D., Manicavasagar V. (2000) *Overcoming Panic: A Self-Help Guide Using Cognitive Behavioural Techniques* (2nd edn). Robinson, London.

De Silva P., Rachman S. (2004) *Obsessive Compulsive Disorder: The Facts* (3rd edn). Oxford University Press, Oxford.

Moncrieff J. (2009) *A Straight Talking Introduction To Psychiatric Drugs*. PCCS Books, Ross on Wye.

Index